New Insights into the Future of Pharmacoepidemiology and Drug Safety

Edited by Maria Teresa Herdeiro, Fátima Roque, Adolfo Figueiras and Tânia Magalhães Silva

Published in London, United Kingdom

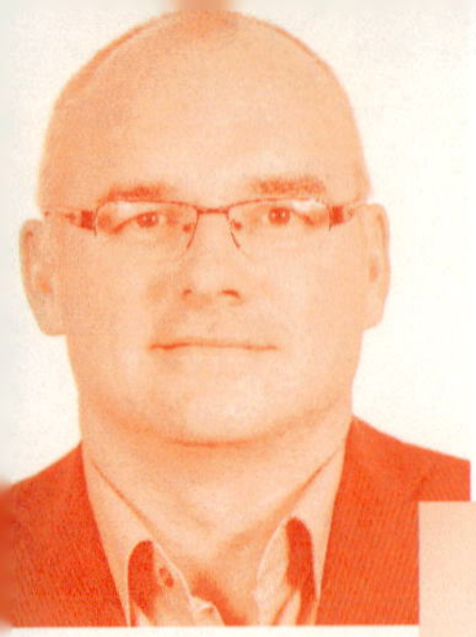
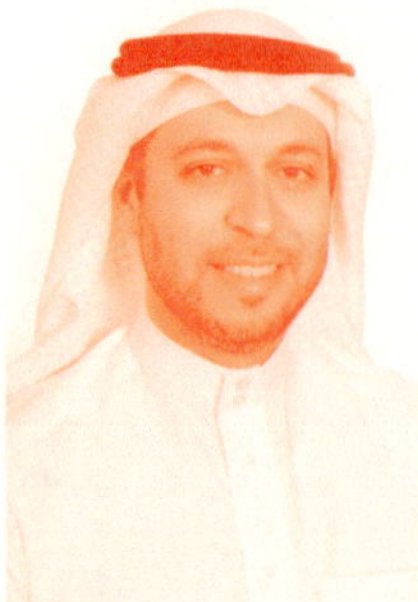
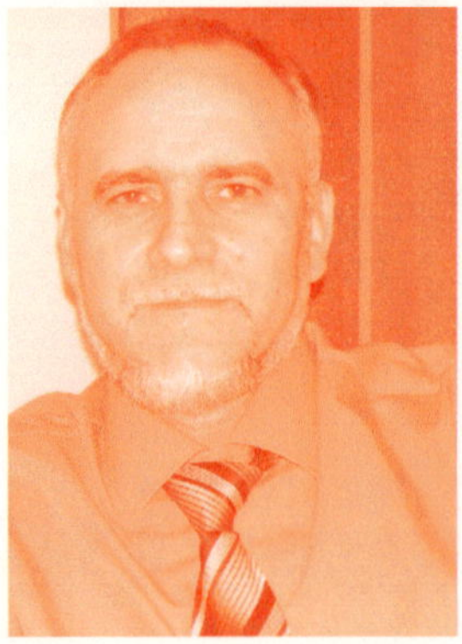
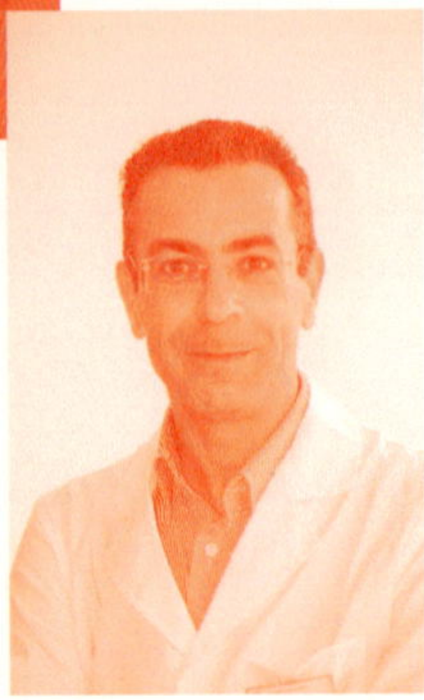
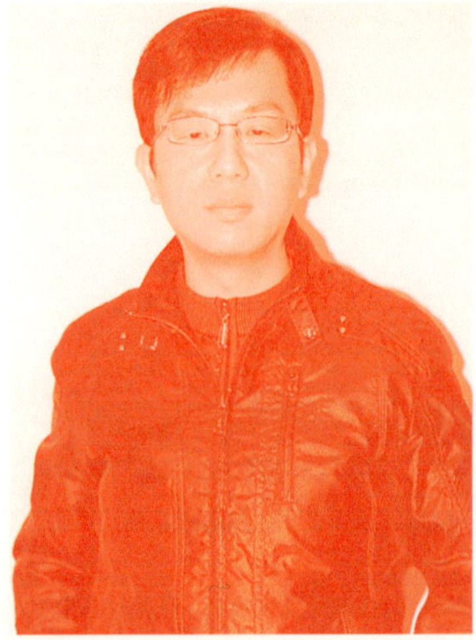
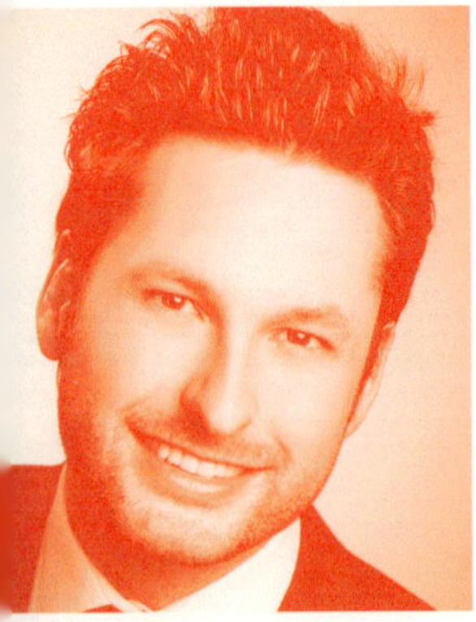
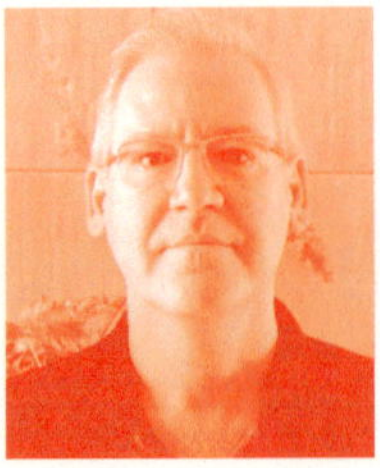

IntechOpen

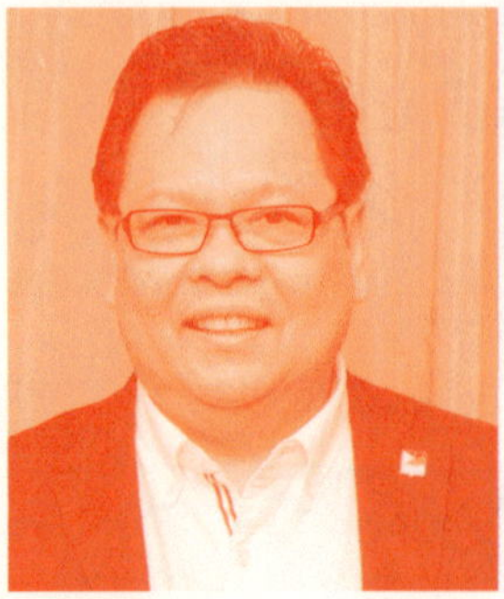
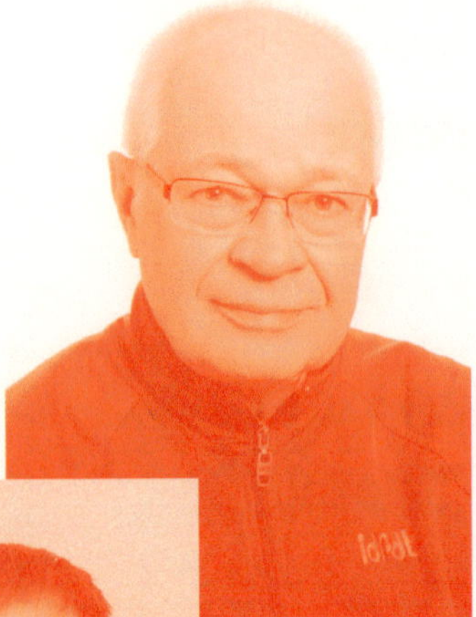
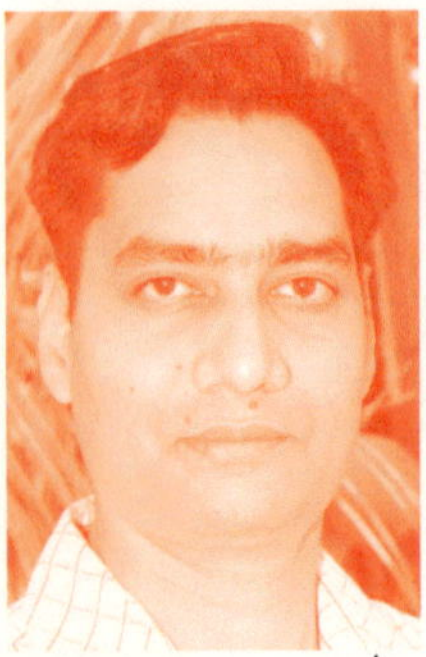
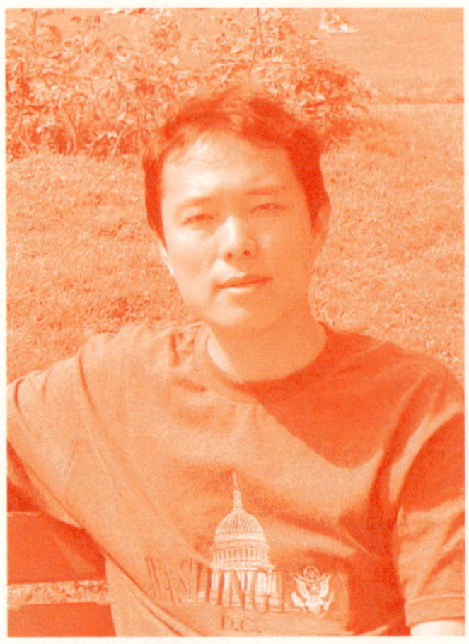
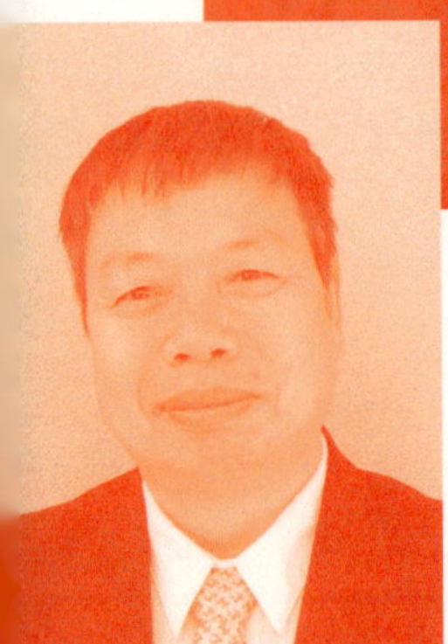
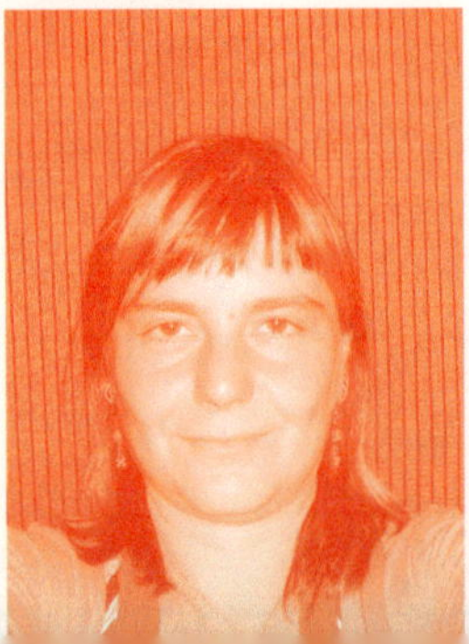

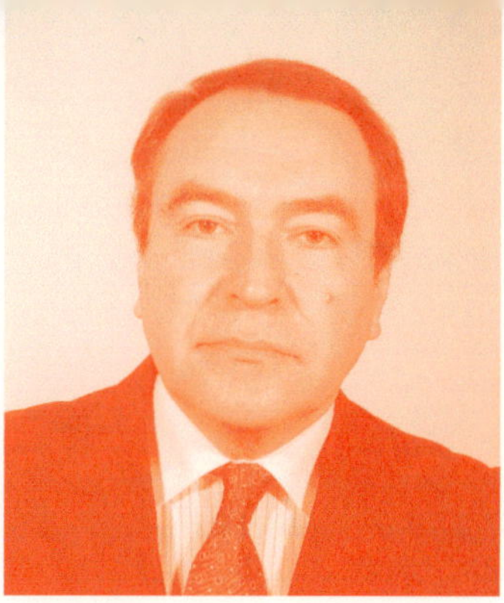
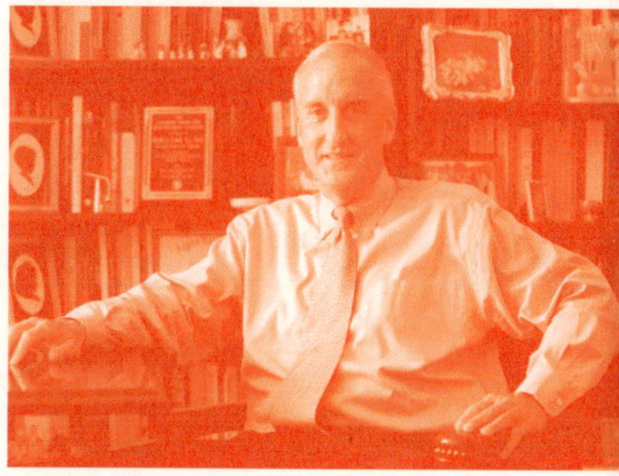
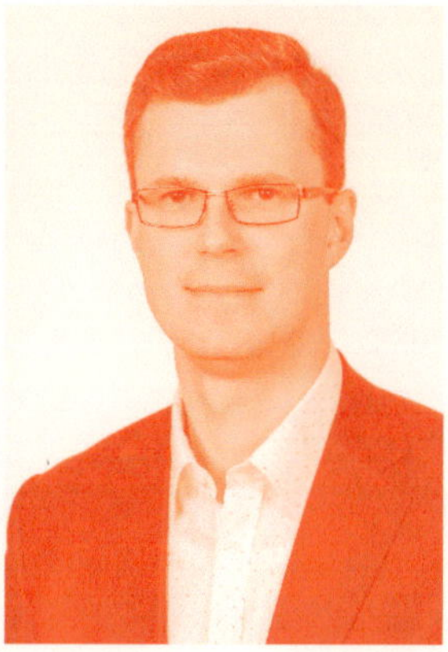
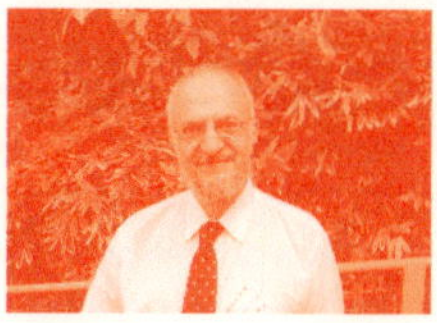
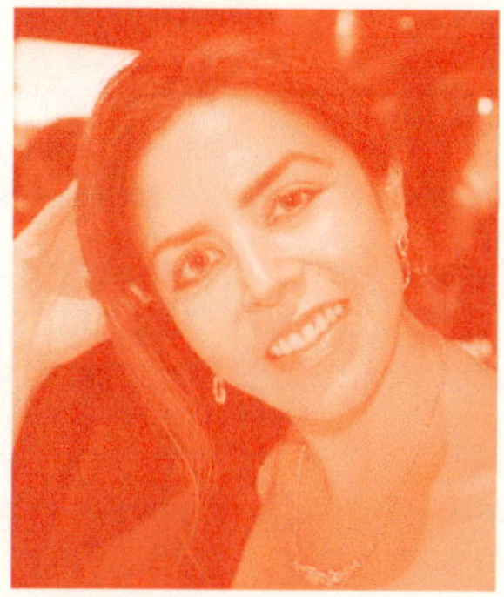

Supporting open minds since 2005

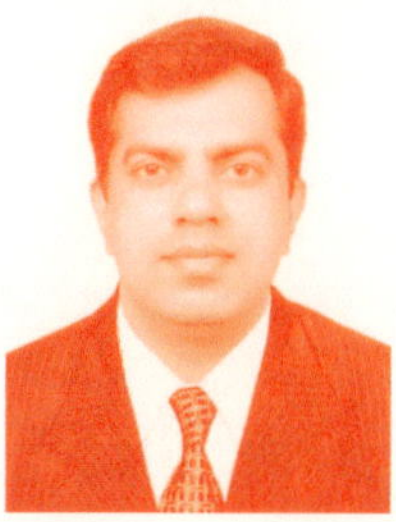
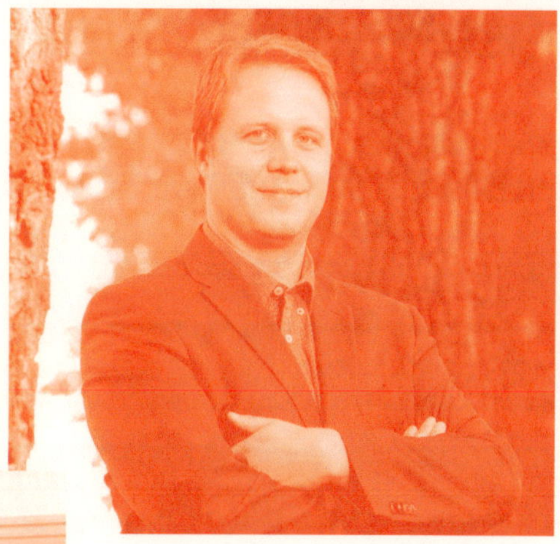
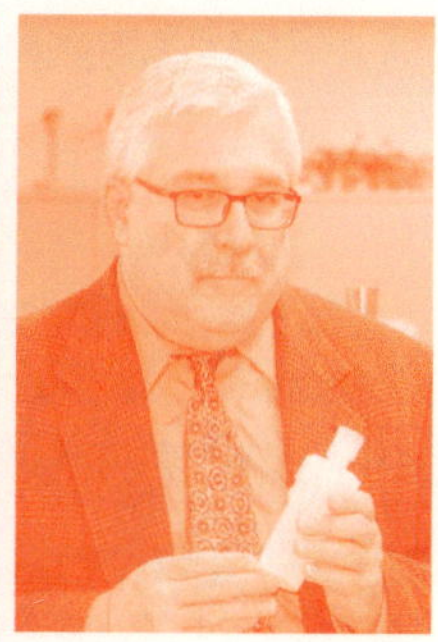
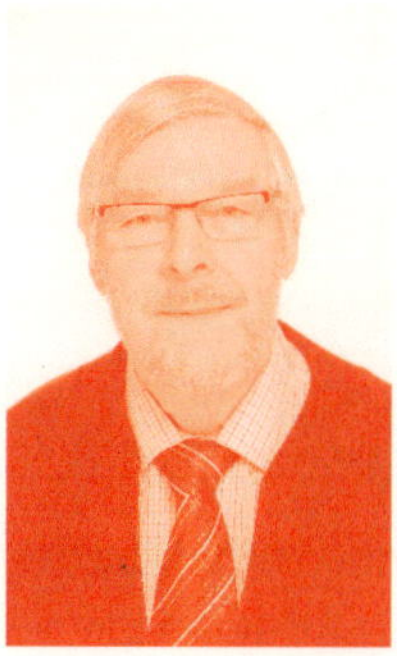
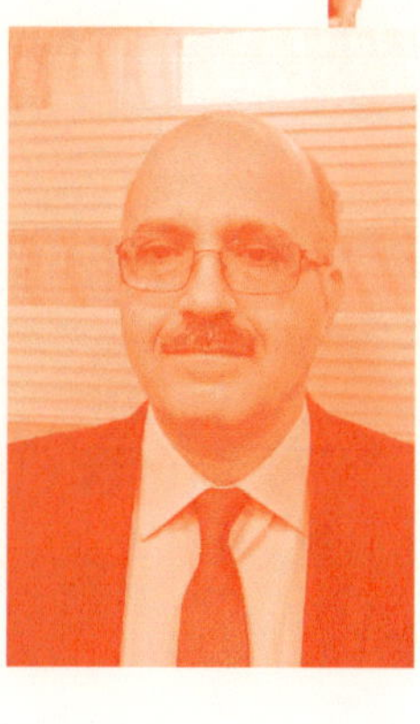
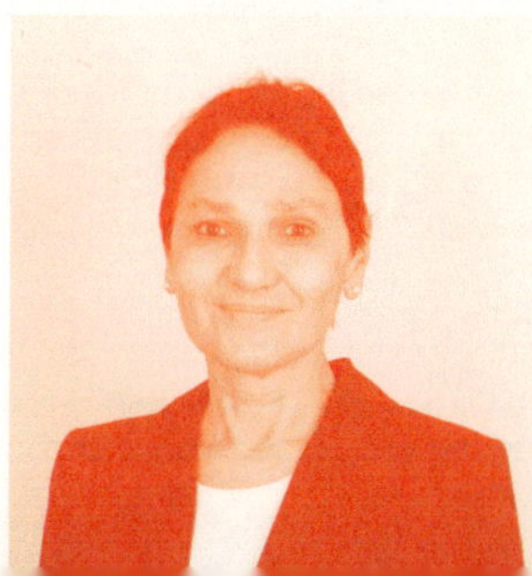
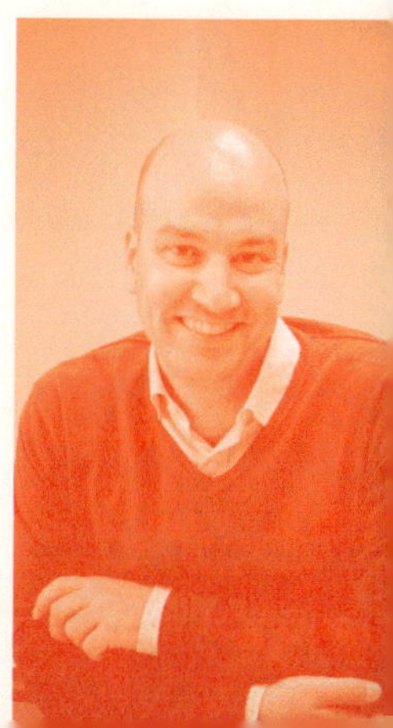

New Insights into the Future of Pharmacoepidemiology and Drug Safety
http://dx.doi.org/10.5772/intechopen.87642
Edited by Maria Teresa Herdeiro, Fátima Roque, Adolfo Figueiras and Tânia Magalhães Silva

Contributors
Vivekanandan Kalaiselvan, Shatrunajay Shukla, S. Ramesh Kumar, Nikita Mishra, Pawan Kumar, Rajeev Singh Raghuvanshi, Shatrunjay Shukla, Ibrahim Chikowe, Elias Peter Mwakilama, Sayna Jabalpeikar, Fabiana Rossi Varallo, Leonardo Régis Leira Pereira, Helaine Carneiro Capucho, Maria Olívia Barboza Zanetti, Ariane Cristina Barboza Zanetti, Vinícius Detoni Lopes, Alan Maicon de Oliveira, Lucas Borges Pereira, Thalita Zago de Oliveira, Fátima Roque, Daniel Gomes, Eva Rebelo Gomes, Inês Ribeiro-Vaz, Maria Teresa Herdeiro, Tânia Magalhães Silva, Md. Shah Amran, Gwendolin S Simper, Gia-Gia Toni Ho, Wiebke Hiemisch, Michelle Matern, Lareen Sophi Gräser, Christina Bade-Doeding, Andreas Pich, Rainer Blasczyk, Adolfo Figueiras

First published in London, United Kingdom, 2021 by IntechOpen
IntechOpen is the global imprint of INTECHOPEN LIMITED, registered in England and Wales, registration number: 11086078, 5 Princes Gate Court, London, SW7 2QJ, United Kingdom
Printed in Croatia

British Library Cataloguing-in-Publication Data
A catalogue record for this book is available from the British Library

Additional hard and PDF copies can be obtained from orders@intechopen.com

New Insights into the Future of Pharmacoepidemiology and Drug Safety
Edited by Maria Teresa Herdeiro, Fátima Roque, Adolfo Figueiras and Tânia Magalhães Silva
p. cm.
Print ISBN 978-1-83968-596-5
Online ISBN 978-1-83968-597-2
eBook (PDF) ISBN 978-1-83968-598-9

Meet the editors

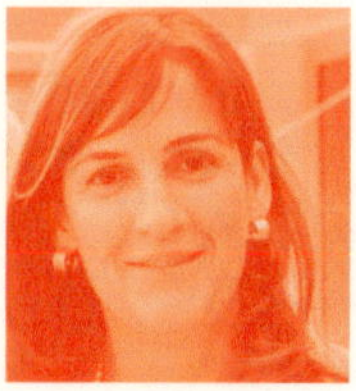

Prof. Dr. Maria Teresa Herdeiro has a Ph.D. in Public Health and Pharmacoepidemiology from the University of Santiago de Compostela, Galicia, Spain. She is a regulatory affairs expert by the Portuguese Pharmacist College and an assistant professor and principal investigator at Aveiro University, Portugal, where she is also a coordinator of the Master's in Clinical Research Management Program. She received the Scientific Research Doctor Odette dos Santos Ferreira award from the Portuguese Pharmacist College in 2012 and the Clinical Epidemiology prize from the Lisbon Society of Medical Sciences and MSD in 2016. Dr. Herdeiro has published more than 60 articles in pharmacovigilance, epidemiology, and public health, and more than 100 oral communications in national and international conferences. She is an editor for six international journals and a member of several financed projects by Fundação para a Ciência e Tecnologia (FCT), Instituto de Salud Carlos III, Conselho Nacional de Desenvolvimento Científico e Tecnológico (CNPq), and Quadro de Referência Estratégico Nacional (QREN).

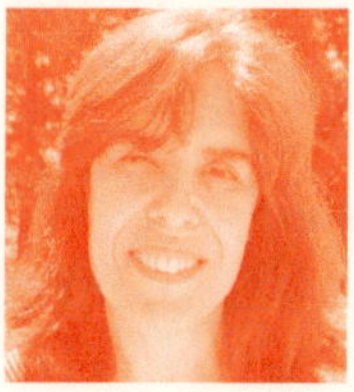

Prof. Dr. Fátima Roque has a Ph.D. in Pharmaceutical Sciences. She is an adjunct professor at the School of Health Sciences, Polytechnic Institute of Guarda, Portugal, and a researcher at the Health Sciences Research Center, University of Beira Interior, Portugal. Dr. Roque is a regulatory affairs expert by Portuguese Pharmacist College. Her research interests include clinical pharmacy, pharmacoepidemiology, and public health. She was awarded the Clinical Epidemiology prize from the Lisbon Society of Medical Sciences and MSD in 2016. She is editor and referee for international journals, as well as the author of more than 40 papers and book chapters in the fields of pharmacoepidemiology and public health, and more than 100 conference communications. Dr. Roque is a member of financed projects by Fundação para a Ciência e Tecnologia (FCT).

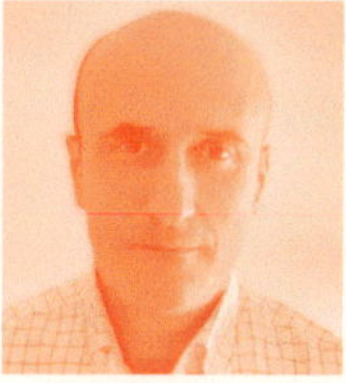

Prof. Dr. Adolfo Figueiras has a degree in Pharmacy, a Ph.D. in Medicine, and a master's in Public Health from the University of Santiago de Compostela, Galicia, Spain, and a master's in Pharmacoepidemiology from the Autonomous University of Barcelona. He is a group leader of the Center for Biomedical Research (CIBER) in Epidemiology and Public Health, coordinator of the Epidemiology, Public Health and Evaluation of Health Services group of the Health Research Institute of Santiago de Compostela (IDIS), and coordinator of the Public Health Master's Degree Program, University of Santiago de Compostela. Dr. Figueiras has more than 100 publications in the fields of epidemiology and public health, has conducted nine projects of the Spanish National Research Plan, and directed fourteen doctoral theses. He has four first prizes from the Spanish Society of Epidemiology, the Spanish Society of Primary Care Pharmacists, and the fourth edition of the Esteves awards.

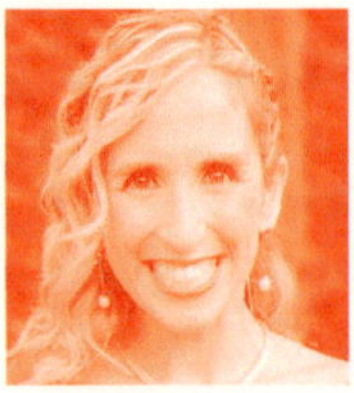

Dr. Tânia Magalhães Silva is a biochemist with a Ph.D. in Biochemistry, with a specialization in Molecular/Cell Biology, from the University of Coimbra, Portugal, and Lund University, Sweden. She has postdocs in Microbiology and Immunology of Infection, and Cell Division, both from the Institute for Molecular and Cellular Biology (IBMC)/i3S, Porto University, Portugal. Dr. Silva was Assistant Professor of Biochemistry and Microbiology at ESSNorte–CVP, Oliveira de Azeméis, and Cell Culture Laboratory Assistant Professor at Lund University. She is currently a junior researcher at iBiMED, Aveiro University, with expertise in biomedical/health sciences, pharmacoepidemiology, clinical research, and public health. She has published more than twelve papers in indexed journals and two book chapters. She has also presented more than thirty oral/poster communications at national and international conferences. Dr. Silva is co-editor of several books published by IntechOpen, a referee of four international journals, and a team member of several financed research projects over the last ten years.

Contents

Preface

Pharmacoepidemiology is a relevant emerging field that applies epidemiological methodologies to study the interactions between health products and large human populations in real-life settings, namely the effects, benefits, and risks of drug use, with the goal of endorsing/optimizing their rational use to improve health outcomes. Pharmacovigilance, or drug safety, is a significant area within pharmacoepidemiology, and addresses the assessment, detection, monitoring, and prevention of adverse drug reactions, thus being fundamental for recognizing the safety of medicines and, at the same time, preventing patients from potential harms.

New Insights into the Future of Pharmacoepidemiology and Drug Safety provides scientific information on important subjects within the fields of pharmacoepidemiology, pharmacovigilance, and drug safety, aiming to improve public health surveillance and shed light on some critical unexplored concepts. Furthermore, it allows readers to acquire an in-depth understanding of the main roles, key principles, developments, and practices adopted in these disciplines while also highlighting their latest advances. This book is for students and those working in pharmacology, epidemiology, drug safety, clinical research, regulatory affairs, pharmacovigilance, and risk management, including researchers, health professionals, and employees from clinical research organizations.

The book contains ten chapters divided into four sections. The introductory chapter "Pharmacovigilance and Public Health Safety" offers a comprehensive overview of the key features of pharmacovigilance and its high importance in preserving public health by enhancing patient safety and quality of life. The remaining nine chapters are included in the following sections.

Section 2, "Recent Findings and New Advances of Adverse Drug Reactions," includes the following five chapters: "Adverse Drug Reactions and Pharmacovigilance," "Adverse Drug Reactions Associated with Anti-Tuberculosis Therapy," "Prevalence and Significance of Antibiotic-Associated Adverse Reactions," "Evaluation of the Medication Safety of Chemotherapy Drugs," and "Small Molecule/HLA Complexes Alter the Cellular Proteomic Content." These chapters explore the significant benefits of monitoring and reporting adverse drug reactions while a drug is in clinical trials as well as after its market authorization. Drugs examined include those used for anti-tuberculosis therapy and chemotherapy as well as antibiotics. Furthermore, this section also reviews the epidemiological data related to antibiotic-associated adverse reactions and analyzes drug–protein interactions within the human leukocyte antigen (HLA) system and its association with adverse drug reactions and disease.

Section 3, "Drug Safety among Older People," includes the two chapters: "Pharmacovigilance in Older Adults" and "Drug-Induced Delirium among Older People." These chapters study the interactions between polypharmacy and adverse drug effects in older adults, such as delirium, namely through the prescription of inappropriate medication, thus highlighting the importance of encouraging pharmacovigilance practices among this special population.

Section 4, "Scientific Methods and Tools for Safety Surveillance" includes two chapters: "Computer-Aided Pharmacoepidemiology in Drug Use and Safety: Examining the Intersection between Data Science and Medicines Research" and "Basics and Essentials of Medical Devices Safety Surveillance." These chapters explore the increasing use of real-world data in pharmacoepidemiologic research and medication safety, while at the same time assessing the main strengths and limitations of relevant healthcare tools such as electronic databases and medical devices.

In sum, this book provides a general overview of past and new scientific research developments in pharmacoepidemiology and drug safety, as well as reinforces the main goals, strengths, and limitations of the most critical concepts within these fields.

Maria Teresa Herdeiro and Tânia Magalhães Silva
iBiMED – Institute of Biomedicine,
Department of Medical Sciences,
University of Aveiro,
Aveiro, Portugal

Fátima Roque
Research Unit for Inland Development – Guarda Polytechnic Institute (UDI-IPG),
Guarda, Portugal

Health Sciences Research Centre,
University of Beira Interior (CICS-UBI),
Covilhã, Portugal

Adolfo Figueiras
Health Research Institute of Santiago de Compostela (IDIS),
University of Santiago de Compostela,
Santiago de Compostela, Spain

Consortium for Biomedical Research in Epidemiology and Public Health
(CIBER Epidemiology and Public Health - CIBERESP),
Madrid, Spain

Section 1

Introduction

Chapter 1

Introductory Chapter: Pharmacovigilance and Public Health Safety

Maria Teresa Herdeiro, Tânia Magalhães Silva, Inês Ribeiro-Vaz, Eva Rebelo Gomes, Adolfo Figueiras and Fátima Roque

1. Introduction to pharmacovigilance

Worldwide, pharmacovigilance is one of the most important scientific disciplines within public health [1]. According to the World Health Organization (WHO), pharmacovigilance is described as "the science and activities relating to the detection, assessment, understanding and prevention of adverse effects or any other drug-related problem" [2]. The implementation of pharmacovigilance activities was essential to globally promote and protect public health, particularly by reducing the significant burden of morbidity, mortality and associated increased healthcare costs, triggered by the occurrence of adverse reactions to medicines [3]. The Memo/08/782, released in 2008 by the European Commission, highlights the importance of pharmacovigilance, namely for saving lives, by revealing estimates of about 197 thousand deaths per year and total costs to society of 79 billion euros in the European Union (EU), due to adverse reactions [4].

The fundamental goals of pharmacovigilance are [5–7]:

- To early identify drug-related problems, such as the occurrence of adverse reactions and other interactions previously unrecognized, reporting the resulting outcomes in a timely manner;

- To detect changes in the incidence of known adverse reactions;

- To carefully monitor and assess the benefit, harm, side-effects, efficacy and risks, together with the risk–benefit profile, of commercialized medicines, aiming to reduce their risks and increase their benefits during the drug's lifecycle;

- To boost the prudent, rational and more effective (including cost-effective) use of several drugs;

- To strengthen patient's care and safety, and consequently safeguard public health, concerning the use of medicines, including paramedical interventions;

- To promote education, knowledge, accurate information and clinical training in the field of drug safety and ensure its effective communication and accessibility to the public.

IntechOpen

In sum, the golden objective of pharmacovigilance process is to enhance patient's safety and quality of life, and strictly preserve public health by identifying, preventing or decreasing the harmful effects and risks related to the use of health products in humans. Therefore, the science that assesses drug's safety and efficacy profiles stands as highly important throughout the entire drug development lifecycle, from preclinical development until post-market surveillance, as it promotes the continuous vigilance of the drug effects. It plays a crucial role within pharmaceuticals, not only for the prevention of drug-related risks in humans, as well as for the reduction of the financial expenses linked to the occurrence of unexpected adverse effects [5–8].

2. Pharmacovigilance history

Pharmacovigilance has a long history. Although the first findings were dated from 172 years ago, when a patient died after being anesthetized with chloroform, followed by 107 deaths in the United States of America in 1937, due to the high toxicity caused by diethyleneglycol, a sulfanilamide elixir-containing solvent, its official inception to address drug safety problems was only heralded after the thalidomide tragedy, in 1961 [1, 8]. This drug was commonly used in Europe by pregnant women as a nonaddictive, nonbarbiturate sedative for nausea treatment, and resulted into a devasting 10 thousand birth abnormalities, namely phocomelia, and increased miscarriage rates [9]. At that time, Dr. McBride highlighted the link between the consumption of thalidomide in pregnancy and the prevalence of fetal congenital malformations, by writing a letter to The Lancet journal editor and reporting an increase of 20% in these cases. In response to the thalidomide disaster, it became evident the urgency in requiring the rigorous safety and efficacy testing of drugs before their market authorization, as well as a global awareness concerning the need for creating pharmacovigilance systems [8].

The pharmacovigilance system suffered many alterations since then and, due to a collaborative effort of many stakeholders, such as physicians, pharmacists, other healthcare professionals, patients, regulatory health authorities, academia and industry, in 1968 the WHO Pilot Research Programme for International Drug Monitoring was instituted. This program intended to establish an active, systematic, organized and regulated network at an international level, mainly for uncovering formerly unknown or poorly recognized drug's adverse effects, leading to the formal adoption of the pharmacovigilance term in the 1970s [7, 8]. In early 1980s, the Council for International Organizations of Medical Sciences (CIOMS) introduced its programme on drug development and usage, together with WHO. In the 1990s, a remarkable impact on international drug regulatory activity was observed, specifically after the implementation of various of the recommendations provided by CIOMS by the formerly International Conference on Harmonization (ICH), currently known as International Council for Harmonization [1, 7, 8]. The ICH helped to harmonize the regulatory infrastructures of the regulatory agencies and pharmaceutical companies from Europe, Japan and the United States [1]. Thereafter, a positive development was observed in several countries, concerning the organization and associated regulations of drug safety, ultimately resulting in the creation of the European Society of Pharmacovigilance (ESOP) in 1992, posteriorly renamed to International Society of Pharmacovigilance (ISoP). Finally, in 1995 the European Medicines Agency (EMA) was founded, followed by the Eudravigilance launch in 2001 [7, 8].

Besides thalidomide disaster, another significant landmark in the history of pharmacovigilance was the market authorization of rofecoxib, a cyclooxigenase-2 inhibitor. In the end of 2000, the Vioxx Gastrointestinal Outcomes Research (VIGOR) study revealed an association between rofecoxib consumption and myocardial infections in patients with chronic pain [10–12]. By this time, this risk became a critical public health issue as rofecoxib was prescribed to tens of millions of people in more than 80 countries. This was one of the most highly publicized drug withdrawals ever reported and, together with other subsequent related episodes, raised some concerns regarding public trust on the role of pre- and post-marketing surveillance [10–13]. Due to the public's lack of confidence on pharmacovigilance, more robust regulations had to be adopted [12, 14]. These include, for instance, the EU risk management plan, implemented in 2005, which became a mandatory document for marketing authorization applications to evaluate the information on drug toxicology, the request for a pharmacovigilance plan as well as for epidemiological information on the population receiving the drug therapy, and the submission of protocols to the regulatory authorities prior to the study start for a proper safety assessment [12]. Other important measures implemented were the education of physicians and medical students, active participation of other health professionals (pharmacists, nurses) in adverse drug reaction (ADR) reporting, feedback transmission and improvements on ADR reporting [14]. The introduction of all these approaches were essential to safeguard public health, with the particularity of primarily assessing the effects on the population, especially on the patient, rather than over the drug under study [6, 12].

3. Pharmacovigilance systems

Given the high importance of pharmacovigilance, currently, countless countries around the world already have well-established, active and robust national pharmacovigilance systems to safeguard patient's wellbeing.

Pharmacovigilance activities of these systems can also involve the [1]:

1. establishment of the safety profile through data collection and management on the drug's safety;

2. analysis of individual case reports to identify early signals of potential drug-related security problems;

3. dynamic risk management to prevent the emergence of potential associated harmful risks following drug's use; and.

4. information transmission to stakeholders and patients.

Therefore, it is not surprising that the WHO programme, responsible to aid in the design, development and assistance of the pharmacovigilance systems, has already 170 countries as partnership members [15].

3.1 WHO collaborating Center for International Drug Monitoring: the Uppsala monitoring Center

As previously referred, the WHO Programme for International Drug Monitoring started, in 1968, to systematically collect all available information on drug's adverse effects, as a worldwide response to the thalidomide disaster. Ten years later, in 1978, with the intuit to support this programme, the Uppsala Monitoring Center (UMC) was set up. The UMC is an international, independent and non-profit center in

Uppsala, Sweden, devoted to investigating the harms and benefits of medicines, to ensure a safe and efficient consumption of these drugs by patients [5, 7].

The key mission of UCM, on behalf of the WHO, is to protect patients through an effective and global pharmacovigilance practice, namely the management of the international database of ADR reports received from each country national center, within the WHO's global pharmacovigilance network [5, 7]. This distinctive WHO data repository, known as VigiBase, is the world's single largest database system of individual case safety reports (ICSR), which are solely submitted by members of the WHO programme [16]. The ICSR, also commonly recognized as "spontaneous" or voluntary ADR report, is a safety document that includes the information needed to support the reporting of adverse events, as well as of products-related problems and consumer complaints generated during the drug post-marketing phase. An ICSR can be filled either in paper or electronically and, to be considered as valid, has to include at least the following four elements: an identifiable patient, one identifiable reporter, one suspected medicinal product and one suspected adverse event [17, 18].

In sum, firstly the national pharmacovigilance system of each country receives the spontaneous ADR reports from health professionals, consumers and pharmaceutical companies. Afterwards, the ICSR are locally validated and evaluated, and a regulatory action can be potentially initiated, if needed. Finally, all the member countries are committed to disclose the on-time reports comprising complete post-marketing data into VigiBase, therefore enabling the uncovering of ADR-associated signs between different countries.

Until May 2019, VigiBase has held over 20 million of ICSR associated with medicines [16]. VigiBase collects the reports sent by the member countries of the WHO program, including 140 full member countries and 30 associate members [19]. The majority of the national joining centers have a straightforward electronic access to these standardized and structured reports, which contain a specific hierarchical code for the particular ADR registered, aiming to help in the fast identification of signals by any country member [5, 7]. The terminologies established for coding adverse reaction terms within the WHO programme, such as the WHO – Adverse Reaction Terminology (WHO-ART), afterwards replaced by the Medical Dictionary for Regulatory Activities (MedDRA), have been broadly embraced by national centers, manufacturers and medicinal product regulators [5, 7].

Spontaneous reporting systems are indispensable to post-marketing surveillance, and have shown to be effective in detecting various types of ADR, especially rare ones. Moreover, the ADR report method also evaluates the need to pursuit further investigations to check if exists an association with the medicine and can hence trigger alarm signals [20]. However, the search for complements to the existing pharmacovigilance systems has shown to be extremely important, mainly due to the significant delays encountered on the detection of more common types of ADR, in addition to the persisting high amount of unreported ADR [20].

3.2 European Medicines Agency

Globally, it is possible to find a selection of regulatory authorities whose main function is to regulate and support pharmacovigilance. For instance, while in the United States, the responsible structure is the Food and Drug Administration (FDA), in the EU is the EMA [21].

Briefly, EMA's gold mission relies on the promotion of scientific merit pertaining to medicine's evaluation and oversight, for the benefit of public and animal health in the EU. In compliance with the EU legislation requirements, EMA's main responsibilities are related to the:

1. supply and communication of independent science-based recommendations concerning the quality, safety and efficacy of medicinal products, especially when highly important to public health safeguard;

2. implementation of measures for continuous control of the quality, safety and efficacy of legalized drugs, namely by guaranteeing a positive benefit/risk ratio;

3. publication of unbiased and reliable information on medicinal products; and

4. development of good practices for drug assessment and regulation in Europe, together with the promotion of harmonized international regulatory standards [21, 22].

The legal pharmacovigilance framework for human medicines marketed within the EU/European Economic Area (EEA) is given in Regulation (EC) No 726/2004, with regard to the EU authorized medicinal products, and Directive 2001/83/EC, concerning the nationally authorized medicinal products, together with the Commission Implementing Regulation (EU) No 520/2012, which summarizes the practical aspects and obligations to be respected and followed by marketing authorization holders and regulatory authorities. Posteriorly, the Directive 2010/84/EC was introduced to substitute the previous directive, with minor amendments being performed in 2012. The EU law requires marketing authorization holders, national competent authorities and EMA to operate services and processes in line with EU legislation, aiming to support a quality assured EU regulatory pharmacovigilance system and to reduce the number of ADR in EU [21–23]. The EU pharmacovigilance system is one of the most sophisticated and comprehensive in the world and allows monitoring the safety of medicines on the European market through prevention, detection and assessment of adverse reactions to drugs, leading to an increased level of public health protection throughout the EU. This system operates through a robust and close collaboration between the competent regulatory authorities from the EU member states, EMA (system coordinator responsible for centrally authorized drugs) and the European Commission (competent authority for drugs centrally authorized in the EU), to rapidly manage and act against an emerging problem, unceasingly prioritizing a safer and more efficacious access of patients to medicinal products. The Pharmacovigilance Risk Assessment Committee (PRAC) was formed in response to this need in July 2012, thus being responsible to provide recommendations on all aspects related to human drugs risk management [21–23].

The European pharmacovigilance network not only successfully collaborates at the European level with high transparency, but also coordinates the necessary regulatory actions, hence producing efficient and accurate safety results able to be transmitted to the EU public in a timely manner. Some of the regulatory tools accessible after the implementation of the revised legislation involve risk management planning, signal detection and management at EU level, periodic safety update reports assessment, drug reviews through referrals post-authorization safety and efficacy studies, communication and training [23].

Within EU, the implementation of the different national pharmacovigilance systems occurred at distinct times. In 1963, The Netherlands became the first EU country to launch their own pharmacovigilance system for spontaneous ADR reporting, followed by the United Kingdom, in 1964, via the Yellow Card Scheme [24].

To achieve a consistent pharmacovigilance system, it is imperative that guidelines and standards are established as they clarify the practical details of the intended information flow, thus being very valuable, for instance, for health professionals training [5]. Thereby, the pharmacovigilance legislation in force in EU since

July 2012 led to the development of an important set of principles and measures on Good Pharmacovigilance Practices (GVP), to conduct the safety monitoring of medicines in EU [25]. One of the EMA's advisors on the development of these guidelines and standards on operational features of the EU pharmacovigilance is PRAC [22]. The GVP guidelines, covering medicinal products authorized in the EU either centrally via EMA or nationally, apply to EU marketing authorization holders, EMA and the competent authorities from each member state. The GVP can slightly differ between countries, thus being established by each country regulatory authorities. Moreover, the guidelines set is divided into two chapter types [25]:

I. major *Pharmacovigilance Processes* (with each module referring only to one distinct process); and

II. *Product- or Population-specific Considerations* (includes vaccines, biological medicinal products and the pediatric population).

Although EMA is known to support several pharmacovigilance databases, the network system used for collecting, managing and analyzing suspected ADR related to authorized medicines within EEA is EudraVigilance. This electronic reporting database system allows the early detection of potential safety signals of post-marketed drugs by effectively analyzing the spontaneous reports previously submitted by marketing authorization holders and member states [26].

The **Figure 1** below synthesizes the key features of pharmacovigilance for the global protection of the public health.

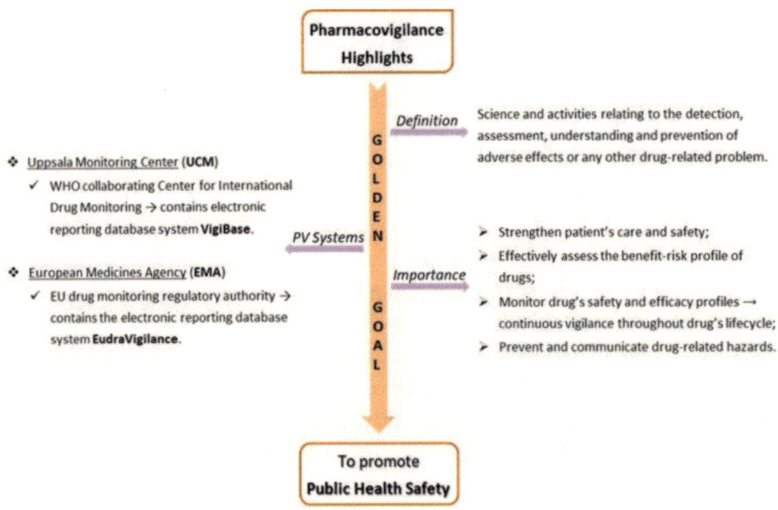

Figure 1.
Pharmacovigilance (PV) highlights in public health safety.

Appendices and nomenclature

ADR	Adverse Drug Reaction
CIOMS	Council for International Organizations of Medical Sciences
EEA	European Economic Area
EMA	European Medicines Agency
ESOP	European Society of Pharmacovigilance

EU	European Union
FDA	Food and Drug Administration
GVP	Good Pharmacovigilance Practices
ICH	International Council for Harmonization
ICSR	Individual Case Safety Report
ISoP	International Society of Pharmacovigilance
MedDRA	Medical Dictionary for Regulatory Activities
PRAC	Pharmacovigilance Risk Assessment Committee
UCM	Uppsala Monitoring Center
VIGOR	Vioxx Gastrointestinal Outcomes Research
WHO	World Health Organization
WHO-ART	World Health Organization-Adverse Reaction Terminology

Author details

Maria Teresa Herdeiro[1*], Tânia Magalhães Silva[1], Inês Ribeiro-Vaz[2,3], Eva Rebelo Gomes[4], Adolfo Figueiras[5,6] and Fátima Roque[7,8]

1 iBiMED - Institute of Biomedicine, Department of Medical Sciences, University of Aveiro, Aveiro, Portugal

2 Porto Pharmacovigilance Center, Faculty of Medicine of University of Porto, Porto, Portugal

3 Center for Health Technology and Services Research (CINTESIS), Faculty of Medicine of University of Porto, Porto, Portugal

4 Allergy and Clinical Immunology Service, University Hospital Center of Porto, Porto, Portugal

5 Department of Preventive Medicine and Public Health, University of Santiago de Compostela, Consortium for Biomedical Research in Epidemiology and Public Health (CIBER en Epidemiología y Salud Pública - CIBERESP), Santiago de Compostela, Spain

6 Health Research Institute of Santiago de Compostela (IDIS), Santiago de Compostela, Spain

7 Research Unit for Inland Development, Guarda Polytechnic Institute (UDI-IPG), Guarda, Portugal

8 Health Sciences Research Center, University of Beira Interior (CICS-UBI), Covilhã, Portugal

*Address all correspondence to: teresaherdeiro@ua.pt

References

[1] Beninger P. Pharmacovigilance: An Overview. Clin Ther [Internet]. 2018 Dec;40(12):1991-2004. Available from: https://linkinghub.elsevier.com/retrieve/pii/S0149291818303175

[2] World Health Organization. Pharmacovigilance: Ensuring the Safe Use of Medicines. [Internet]. Geneva, WHO; 2004 [cited 2020 Nov 7]. Available from: www.who.int/medicines/areas/quality_safety/safety_efficacy/pharmvigi/en/

[3] Santoro A, Genov G, Spooner A, Raine J, Arlett P. Promoting and Protecting Public Health: How the European Union Pharmacovigilance System Works. Drug Saf [Internet]. 2017 Oct 22;40(10):855-69. Available from: http://link.springer.com/10.1007/s40264-017-0572-8

[4] European Commission. MEMO/08/782: Strengthening pharmacovigilance to reduce adverse effects of medicines. [Internet]. Brussels; 2008. Available from: https://ec.europa.eu/commission/presscorner/detail/en/MEMO_08_782

[5] WHO. The Safety of Medicines in Public Health Programmes: Pharmacovigilance an essential tool [Internet]. WHO Collaborating Centre for International Drug Monitoring; 2006. Available from: https://www.who.int/hiv/pub/pharmacovigilance/safety/en/

[6] Pitts PJ, Louet H Le, Moride Y, Conti RM. 21st century pharmacovigilance: efforts, roles, and responsibilities. Lancet Oncol [Internet]. 2016 Nov;17(11):e486-92. Available from: https://linkinghub.elsevier.com/retrieve/pii/S1470204516303126

[7] WHO. The Importance of Pharmacovigilance: Safety Monitoring of medicinal products [Internet]. WHO Collaborating Centre for International Drug Monitoring; 2002. Available from: https://apps.who.int/iris/handle/10665/42493

[8] Fornasier G, Francescon S, Leone R, Baldo P. An historical overview over Pharmacovigilance. Int J Clin Pharm [Internet]. 2018 Aug 15;40(4):744-7. Available from: http://link.springer.com/10.1007/s11096-018-0657-1

[9] Kim JH, Scialli AR. Thalidomide: The Tragedy of Birth Defects and the Effective Treatment of Disease. Toxicol Sci [Internet]. 2011 Jul;122(1):1-6. Available from: https://academic.oup.com/toxsci/article/1672454/Thalidomide:

[10] Waxman HA. The Lessons of Vioxx — Drug Safety and Sales. N Engl J Med [Internet]. 2005 Jun 23;352(25):2576-8. Available from: http://www.nejm.org/doi/abs/10.1056/NEJMp058136

[11] Barry AR, Koshman SL, Pearson GJ. Adverse drug reactions: The importance of maintaining pharmacovigilance. Can Pharm J / Rev des Pharm du Canada [Internet]. 2014 Jul 2;147(4):233-8. Available from: http://journals.sagepub.com/doi/10.1177/1715163514536523

[12] Greener M. First do no harm. EMBO Rep [Internet]. 2008 Mar 8;9(3):221-4. Available from: https://onlinelibrary.wiley.com/doi/abs/10.1038/embor.2008.17

[13] Huybrechts KF, Desai RJ, Park M, Gagne JJ, Najafzadeh M, Avorn J. The Potential Return on Public Investment in Detecting Adverse Drug Effects. Med Care [Internet]. 2017 Jun;55(6):545-51. Available from: http://journals.lww.com/00005650-201706000-00002

[14] Dainesi SM. Pharmacovigilance: more than ever, an overall responsibility. Clinics [Internet].

2005 Aug;60(4). Available from: http://www.scielo.br/scielo.php?script=sci_arttext&pid=S1805932200500040002&lng=en&nrm=iso&tlng=en

[15] Uppsala Monitoring Center [Internet]. [cited 2020 Nov 9]. Available from: https://www.who-umc.org/about-us/who-we-are/

[16] Uppsala Monitoring Centre. VigiBase [Internet]. [cited 2020 Nov 9]. Available from: https://www.who-umc.org/vigibase/vigibase/

[17] Jalali RK. Individual Case Safety Reports. In: Pharmaceutical Medicine and Translational Clinical Research [Internet]. Elsevier; 2018. p. 413-8. Available from: https://linkinghub.elsevier.com/retrieve/pii/B9780128021033000298

[18] European Medicines Agency. Guideline on good pharmacovigilance practices (GVP) Module VI – Collection, management and submission of reports of suspected adverse reactions to medicinal products [Internet]. 2017. Available from: https://www.ema.europa.eu/en/documents/regulatory-procedural-guideline/guideline-good-pharmacovigilance-practices-gvp-module-vi-collection-management-submission-reports_en.pdf

[19] Uppsala Monitoring Center. WHO Programme Members for International Drug Monitoring [Internet]. Available from: https://www.who-umc.org/global-pharmacovigilance/who-programme-for-international-drug-monitoring/who-programme-members/

[20] Baldo P, Francescon S, Fornasier G. Pharmacovigilance workflow in Europe and Italy and pharmacovigilance terminology. Int J Clin Pharm [Internet]. 2018 Aug 9;40(4):748-53. Available from: http://link.springer.com/10.1007/s11096-018-0711-z

[21] Felix T, Jordan JB, Akers C, Patel B, Drago D. Current state of biologic pharmacovigilance in the European Union: improvements are needed. Expert Opin Drug Saf [Internet]. 2019 Mar 4;18(3):231-40. Available from: https://www.tandfonline.com/doi/full/10.1080/14740338.2019.1577818

[22] European Medicines Agency. EMA pharmacovigilance system manual, version 1.2. [Internet]. 2016. Available from: https://www.ema.europa.eu/en/documents/other/european-medicines-agency-pharmacovigilance-system-manual_en.pdf

[23] European Commission. Monitoring safety of medicines for patients. Pharmacovigilance activities related to medicines for human use in the EU [Internet]. 2017. Available from: https://ec.europa.eu/health/sites/health/files/files/pharmacovigilance/pharmacovigilance-report-2012-2014.pdf

[24] Rabbur RSM, Emmerton L. An introduction to adverse drug reaction reporting systems in different countries. Int J Pharm Pract [Internet]. 2005 Mar 1;13(1):91-100. Available from: http://doi.wiley.com/10.1211/0022357055821

[25] European Medicines Agency. Guidelines on good pharmacovigilance practices (GVP) - Introductory cover note [Internet]. 2020. Available from: https://www.ema.europa.eu/en/documents/regulatory-procedural-guideline/guidelines-good-pharmacovigilance-practices-gvp-introductory-cover-note-last-updated-revision-3_en.pdf

[26] Postigo R, Brosch S, Slattery J, van Haren A, Dogné J-M, Kurz X, et al. EudraVigilance Medicines Safety Database: Publicly Accessible Data for Research and Public Health Protection. Drug Saf [Internet]. 2018 Jul 9;41(7):665-75. Available from: http://link.springer.com/10.1007/s40264-018-0647-1

Section 2

Recent Findings and New Advances of Adverse Drug Reactions

Chapter 2

Adverse Drug Reactions and Pharmacovigilance

Md. Shah Amran

Abstract

The discovery of a new drug usually takes 10-15 years. Within this time period, the candidate drug is thoroughly screened for its beneficial as well as side effects. But the side, adverse or toxic effects cannot be detected to a full scale due to some special reasons. The beneficial effects and toxicity of new drugs and vaccines are usually studied by "Clinical trials", which are divided into four categories ranging from clinical trial phases I to IV. During clinical trial phase-III, about 4,000-10,000 patients are involved and after passing this phase, the drug is allowed to enter into the global market. Then, billions of people, including those who were excluded in phase-III, may be administered with this drug. It is worthy to mention that these 4,000-10,000 patients may not show many of the side effects or toxic actions. The undetected adverse drug reactions (ADRs) are studied in clinical trial phase-IV, which is also known as post market surveillance. For this reason, the ADRs are compared with the tip of the iceberg, as it indicates the minor part of a major event. This phenomenon gave birth to a new branch of the pharmacology known as Pharmacovigilance.

Keywords: Adverse drug reaction, Drug safety, Pharmacovigilance, Phocomelia, Post market surveillance

1. Introduction

The discovery of a new drug can usually take 10-15 years [1, 2]. Within this time period, the candidate drug is screened for its beneficial as well as for its side effects (**Figure 1**). But the side, adverse or toxic effects cannot be detected to a full scale due to some special reasons.

Adverse Drug Reaction (ADR) is a damage or injury response caused due to intake of medication [3]. The ADRs may arise after administration of a single dose, or long-term administration of any drug or consequence of the administration of two or more drugs as a combination product or separately [4]. The study of ADRs has turned to be a separate field of science and is known as Pharmacovigilance (PV), which is defined by the World Health Organization (WHO) as, "the science and activities relating to the detection, assessment, understanding and prevention of adverse effects or any other drug-related problem" [5]. The Program for International Drug Monitoring (PIDM) was established by WHO in 1968 in response to the tragedy caused by thalidomide in 1961. The "Thalidomide Tragedy" was related to the birth of children with deformed limbs, also known as phocomelia [6], and it became one of the most known tragedies in the history of medical and pharmaceutical sciences. The WHO encourages, supports and promotes PV at

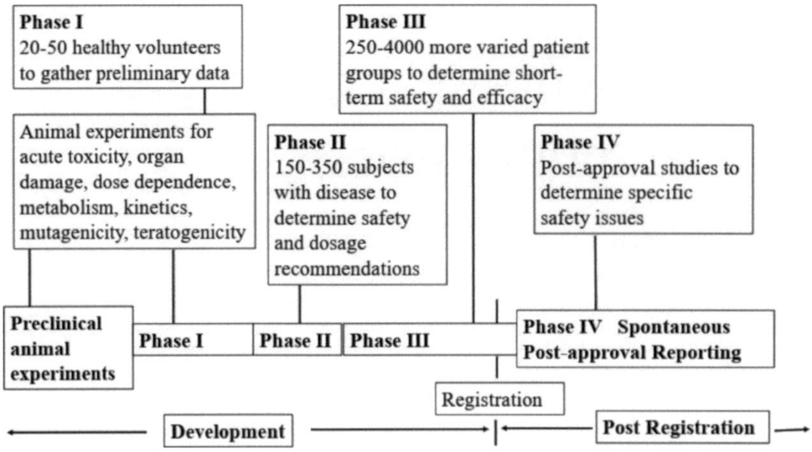

Figure 1.
Steps of drug development and commercialization.

the country level for its member countries, and offers collaboration through its Collaborating Centre for International Drug Monitoring in Uppsala, Sweden [7]. Until March 2019, the total number of member states which have enrolled in the WHO PIDM as a member corresponds to 142 and, additionally 29 associate members are expecting full membership [8].

To prevent tragedies such as the thalidomide disaster, governments all over the world took necessary ethical and legal actions and strengthened their drug regulatory authorities (DRAs) to keep alert and to ensure the marketing of relatively safe drugs.

2. Adverse drug reaction

An ADR can be defined as "any response to a drug which is noxious and unintended, and which occurs at doses used in man for prophylaxis, diagnosis or therapy of disease, or for the modification of physiological function" [9].

2.1 The importance of studying ADRs

As we have mentioned earlier, the overall toxicity of a drug is clearly understood during the whole life cycle of a drug, while only a minor portion of these toxicities are unveiled during clinical trial phases. After global launching, the post market surveillance studies help to assess the information leading to drug withdrawals, safety alerts from regulatory authorities and changes in product labelling. This also triggers the advances in pharmacology and therapeutics. Directly or indirectly, reports of ADR studies have shaped much of the current drug regulatory framework and contributed significantly to drug regulatory decisions. Furthermore, some ADR reports have also proved to be valuable weapons in discoveries in pharmacology and in improving drug use [10]. Clinical trial phases [11] include a small number of population and many clinical trials usually exclude:

1. Children,

2. Old people,

3. Pregnant and lactating women,

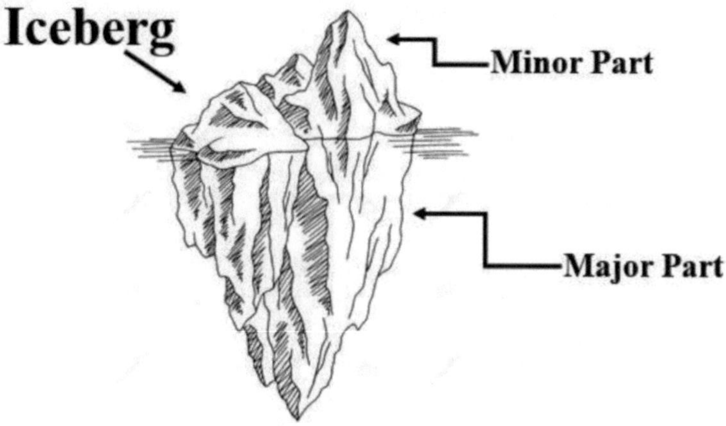

Figure 2.
The schematic diagram of an iceberg [12].

4. Ethnic groups,

5. Peoples with genetic disorders and,

6. People with liver and kidney insufficiency.

During the development of a drug, only less than 50% of ADRs can usually be detected, with the remaining more than 50% being detected after global launching, during the whole life cycle of the product. This can be compared with tip of the iceberg, which indicates a minor part of a major problem (**Figure 2**).

That is why it is very important to study the ADRs after launching of a new drug or vaccine.

3. Drug tragedies abroad and at home

As will be mentioned and described below, the "Thalidomide-induced Phocomelia" led the drug regulatory authority to take rigorous actions, including regulatory actions against the drug and promulgation of regulatory guidelines, as well as legislation. This and other reports have helped to discover a number of major drug disasters, such as the Benoxaprofen (known to cause severe hepatotoxicity and a variety of cutaneous reactions), Torsadogenic Drugs (e.g., prenylamine, terfenadine, cisapride that caused QT prolongation), Practolol (known to cause exfoliative dermatitis, systemic lupus syndrome, drug eruption, psoriasiform eruptions, skin reactions with eye signs consisting of atypical conjunctival shrinkage and xerosis, and keratoconjunctivitis sicca) [10]. In Bangladesh, the "Paracetamol tragedy" led the Directorate General of Drug Administration (DGDA) to take strict regulatory actions in the manufacture and quality control of drugs by the manufacturers. A few examples of those drug tragedies that occurred abroad and in Bangladesh are discussed below.

3.1 The thalidomide tragedy in Europe

In December 1961, William McBride, an Australian obstetrician, alerted in a letter to the *Lancet* that he had seen "multiple severe abnormalities" in babies born from ladies who had been administered with 'thalidomide' at the time of their pregnancy (**Figure 3**) [13]. Dr. McBride summarized his report by questioning if any of their readers had seen similar abnormalities in babies born from women who had taken this drug during pregnancy.

The letter the first printed and published suggestion from a medical doctor about the teratogenic effect of thalidomide in women and it was a brief publication containing only five sentences. Dr. McBride's apprehensions about the drug thalidomide were eventually settled by numerous babies who were born with birth defects [14, 15].

In 2016, a *BMJ* publication about a chronicled film, describing the lives of persons born with birth defects as a consequence of the administration of the medicines narrated, reported the following: "The thalidomide scandal stands as one of the worst ever medical disasters" [16, 17].

3.1.1 Worldwide recognition

William Griffith McBride was born on the 25th of May 1927 in Sydney, Australia. As his mother was sick, he had to spend much of his early living with an aunt on a dairy farm. He pursued his study of medical sciences at Sydney University Medical School.

Dr. McBride attained global recognition for his contribution to alert everyone worldwide about the danger of the drug thalidomide, which have caused defects in the development of the limbs of the fetus and, ultimately, gave rise to the birth of truncated babies. In Australia, his own country, Dr. McBride was praised as a national hero, and a radiance of honor fell over him over the next three decades. He had a blooming practice in Sydney, and he was awarded with both the 'Commander of the Order of the British Empire' in 1969 and the Order of Australia in 1977.

But a later part of McBride's life and work was not so pleasing. In 1993, when he was 65, McBride was found guilty of scientific deception by a medical court for the consciously publishing of erroneous and fallacious research. Consequently, his name was cut from the medical register [18–20].

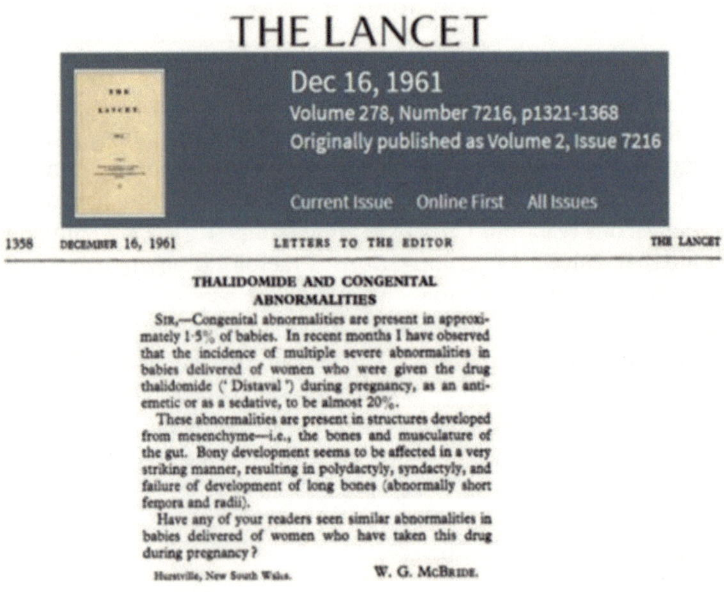
THE LANCET

Dec 16, 1961

Volume 278, Number 7216, p1321-1368

Originally published as Volume 2, Issue 7216

Current Issue Online First All Issues

1358 DECEMBER 16, 1961 LETTERS TO THE EDITOR THE LANCET

THALIDOMIDE AND CONGENITAL ABNORMALITIES

SIR,—Congenital abnormalities are present in approximately 1·5% of babies. In recent months I have observed that the incidence of multiple severe abnormalities in babies delivered of women who were given the drug thalidomide ('Distaval') during pregnancy, as an anti-emetic or as a sedative, to be almost 20%.

These abnormalities are present in structures developed from mesenchyme—i.e., the bones and musculature of the gut. Bony development seems to be affected in a very striking manner, resulting in polydactyly, syndactyly, and failure of development of long bones (abnormally short femora and radii).

Have any of your readers seen similar abnormalities in babies delivered of women who have taken this drug during pregnancy?

Hurstville, New South Wales. W. G. McBRIDE.

Figure 3.
The first page of the letter to the editor published in the scientific journal 'The Lancet', in 1961, on the adverse effects of thalidomide.

3.2 Sulfonamide tragedy in Chicago, USA

An article reporting to the "Sulfanilamide Disaster" was published in June 1981 in an issue from the FDA Consumer magazine, and was entitled "Taste of Raspberries, Taste of Death: The 1937 Elixir Sulfanilamide Incident" [21]. The incident was described as: "By the 1930s it was widely recognized that the Food and Drugs Act of 1906 was obsolete, but bitter disagreement arose as to what should replace it. By 1937 most of the arguments had been resolved but Congressional action was stalled. Then came a shocking development: the deaths of more than 100 people after using a drug that was clearly unsafe. The incident hastened final enactment in 1938 of the Federal Food, Drug, and Cosmetic Act, the statute that today remains the basis for FDA regulation of these products".

Sulfanilamide is used to treat streptococcal infections due to its curative effects and, at that time, was available in the form of tablet and powder dosage. The demand for the liquid dosage form was raised by a salesman of the S.E. Massengill Co., in Bristol, Tenn., and the company's principal chemist and pharmacist, Harold Cole Watkins, who used diethylene glycol to dissolve sulfonamide and prepare an elixir. The quality control laboratory of the company analyzed the product for flavor, appearance and fragrance, and certified it as satisfactory. Instantly, the company considered it as a safe product, manufactured a certain quantity of it and sent product shipments to the whole country [21]. The new dosage form had not been analyzed for its toxicity and no pharmacological evaluation had been performed on the new sulfanilamide preparation. Watkins failed to record one feature of the elixir made by using diethylene glycol, which is applied as an antifreeze and is a lethal poison, causing renal damage followed by death [21].

3.3 Tylenol tragedy

Tylenol (Paracetamol) tragedy occurred in 1982 [22]. Tylenol was a product of of Johnson & Johnson and a trade-named drug intended for lessening pain, decreasing fever, and alleviating the symptoms of cough, cold, headache, allergies and influenza. The active pharmaceutical ingredient of this preparation is paracetamol (in the US it is known as acetaminophen), which is prescribed as an analgesic and antipyretic. The branded name (market name) Tylenol is accrued from a chemical name for the compound, N-acetyl-para-aminophenol (APAP). The branded name is possessed by McNeil Consumer Healthcare [22].

In 1982, in Chicago, US, Tylenol capsules laced with potassium cyanide caused the death of at least seven persons and raised a big concern about the safety of the marketed product. Potassium cyanide looks like normal table sugar, is water soluble but very toxic, being usually used for suicide (it is also known as suicide pills) [23].

This accident guided to the reforms in the packaging of over-the-counter drugs and to central anti-tampering laws. Johnson & Johnson took some necessary actions in their packaging and marketing policy that led to a reduction in the number of deaths and warned the public about potential poisoning risks. This action has been widely glorified as an exemplary public relation response to such a big crisis. Thus, Johnson & Johnson became able to regain their market share, which had been lost due to the Tylenol incident [22–24].

3.4 Paracetamol tragedy in Bangladesh

Two critical mishaps happened with paracetamol in Bangladesh. The first one occurred during 1990 to 1993, with the paracetamol produced by Adflame Pharmaceuticals Limited, and the second one took place during 2009 to 2010, with the paracetamol manufactured by Rid Pharmaceuticals Limited. These two incidents are described below.

i. Adflame Pharmaceuticals Limited (1990 – 1993)

From 1990 to 1992, about 339 children developed renal failure in Bangladesh, and most of them died, after being given paracetamol (acetaminophen) solution using diethylene glycol [25]. The drug was manufactured by the "Adflame Pharmaceuticals Limited", Savar, Dhaka. The incident compelled the national government to forbid the trading of paracetamol preparations. Consequently, a decrease of 53% in the admission of victims with kidney failure and of 84% in admissions by unexplored kidney failure was observed in December 1992. This drug-related accident was reported in BMJ (**Figure 4**) in 1995 [25].

Three persons of the Adflame Pharmaceutical company were given 10-years of rigorous jail for producing a spurious drug which slaughtered 76 children in the 1990s. These convicted persons were Helena Pasha (Director), Mizanur Rahman (Manager) and Nigendra Nath Bala (production officer).

The prosecution against the manufacturing entity Adflame was only one of the four others also involved in this petition. Three other pharmaceutical producers were also accused of manufacturing the same contaminated liquid

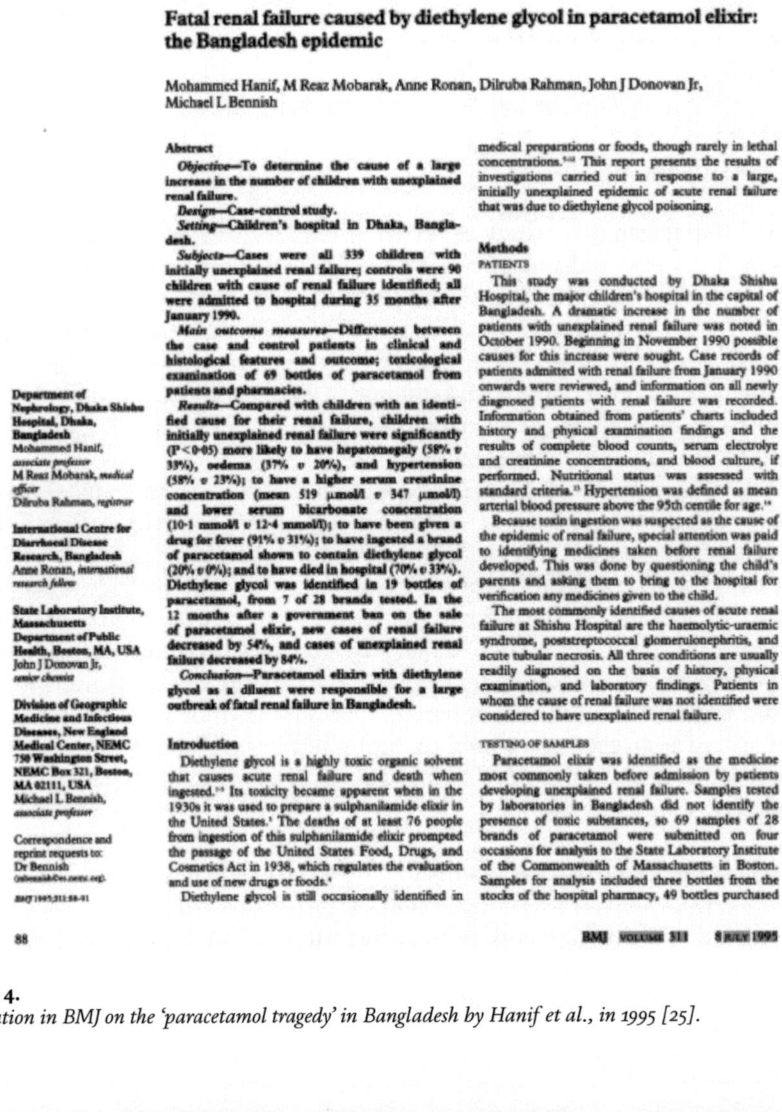

Fatal renal failure caused by diethylene glycol in paracetamol elixir: the Bangladesh epidemic

Mohammed Hanif, M Reaz Mobarak, Anne Ronan, Dilruba Rahman, John J Donovan Jr, Michael L Bennish

Abstract

Objective—To determine the cause of a large increase in the number of children with unexplained renal failure.

Design—Case-control study.

Setting—Children's hospital in Dhaka, Bangladesh.

Subjects—Cases were all 339 children with initially unexplained renal failure; controls were 90 children with cause of renal failure identified; all were admitted to hospital during 35 months after January 1990.

Main outcome measures—Differences between the case and control patients in clinical and histological features and outcome; toxicological examination of 69 bottles of paracetamol from patients and pharmacies.

Results—Compared with children with an identified cause for their renal failure, children with initially unexplained renal failure were significantly ($P<0·05$) more likely to have hepatomegaly (58% v 33%), oedema (37% v 20%), and hypertension (58% v 23%); to have a higher serum creatinine concentration (mean 519 μmol/l v 347 μmol/l) and lower serum bicarbonate concentration (10·1 mmol/l v 12·4 mmol/l); to have been given a drug for fever (91% v 31%); to have ingested a brand of paracetamol shown to contain diethylene glycol (20% v 0%); and to have died in hospital (70% v 33%). Diethylene glycol was identified in 19 bottles of paracetamol, from 7 of 28 brands tested. In the 12 months after a government ban on the sale of paracetamol elixir, new cases of renal failure decreased by 54%, and cases of unexplained renal failure decreased by 84%.

Conclusion—Paracetamol elixirs with diethylene glycol as a diluent were responsible for a large outbreak of fatal renal failure in Bangladesh.

Department of Nephrology, Dhaka Shishu Hospital, Dhaka, Bangladesh
Mohammed Hanif, *associate professor*
M Reaz Mobarak, *medical officer*
Dilruba Rahman, *registrar*

International Centre for Diarrhoeal Disease Research, Bangladesh
Anne Ronan, *international research fellow*

State Laboratory Institute, Massachusetts Department of Public Health, Boston, MA, USA
John J Donovan Jr, *senior chemist*

Division of Geographic Medicine and Infectious Diseases, New England Medical Center, NEMC 750 Washington Street, NEMC Box 321, Boston, MA 02111, USA
Michael L Bennish, *associate professor*

Correspondence and reprint requests to: Dr Bennish

BMJ 1995;311:88-91

Introduction

Diethylene glycol is a highly toxic organic solvent that causes acute renal failure and death when ingested.[1-3] Its toxicity became apparent when in the 1930s it was used to prepare a sulphanilamide elixir in the United States.[3] The deaths of at least 76 people from ingestion of this sulphanilamide elixir prompted the passage of the United States Food, Drugs, and Cosmetics Act in 1938, which regulates the evaluation and use of new drugs or foods.[4]

Diethylene glycol is still occasionally identified in medical preparations or foods, though rarely in lethal concentrations.[5-10] This report presents the results of investigations carried out in response to a large, initially unexplained epidemic of acute renal failure that was due to diethylene glycol poisoning.

Methods

PATIENTS

This study was conducted by Dhaka Shishu Hospital, the major children's hospital in the capital of Bangladesh. A dramatic increase in the number of patients with unexplained renal failure was noted in October 1990. Beginning in November 1990 possible causes for this increase were sought. Case records of patients admitted with renal failure from January 1990 onwards were reviewed, and information on all newly diagnosed patients with renal failure was recorded. Information obtained from patients' charts included history and physical examination findings and the results of complete blood counts, serum electrolye and creatinine concentrations, and blood culture, if performed. Nutritional status was assessed with standard criteria.[13] Hypertension was defined as mean arterial blood pressure above the 95th centile for age.[14]

Because toxin ingestion was suspected as the cause of the epidemic of renal failure, special attention was paid to identifying medicines taken before renal failure developed. This was done by questioning the child's parents and asking them to bring to the hospital for verification any medicines given to the child.

The most commonly identified causes of acute renal failure at Shishu Hospital are the haemolytic-uraemic syndrome, poststreptococcal glomerulonephritis, and acute tubular necrosis. All three conditions are usually readily diagnosed on the basis of history, physical examination, and laboratory findings. Patients in whom the cause of renal failure was not identified were considered to have unexplained renal failure.

TESTING OF SAMPLES

Paracetamol elixir was identified as the medicine most commonly taken before admission by patients developing unexplained renal failure. Samples tested by laboratories in Bangladesh did not identify the presence of toxic substances, so 69 samples of 28 brands of paracetamol were submitted on four occasions for analysis to the State Laboratory Institute of the Commonwealth of Massachusetts in Boston. Samples for analysis included three bottles from the stocks of the hospital pharmacy, 49 bottles purchased

88 BMJ VOLUME 311 8 JULY 1995

Figure 4.
Publication in BMJ on the 'paracetamol tragedy' in Bangladesh by Hanif et al., in 1995 [25].

paracetamol, including Polychem Laboratories Ltd., BCI (Bangladesh) Ltd., and Rex Pharmaceuticals. The fifth pharmaceutical industry - City Chemical and Pharmaceutical Works Ltd., was also sued but not trialed.

ii. Rid Pharmaceuticals Limited, Brahmanbaria (2009–2010)

Once more, in 2009, 28 children died due to the diethylene glycol toxicity [26]. The national government started to constitute a probe committee which detected the presence of the toxic substance diethylene glycol in the liquid paracetamol of one pharmaceutical company, after investigating 300 samples of liquid paracetamol and liquid vitamins of 10 industries. This company was supposed to use propylene glycol, but instead used the toxic diethylene glycol, a component applied in tannery and battery industries. Consequently, its manufactory was completely sealed off and its goods were re-called from the market [26].

In 2016, the drug court (at Dhaka) decided to exonerate all five persons from the Rid Pharmaceutical Industry Ltd., in the case where a poisonous paracetamol was produced and authorized by this company, leading to the death of 28 children all over the country in 2009. The Dhaka drug court judge Mr. Atoar Rahman issued the order on a Monday afternoon. In the verdict, the judge slammed the drug authority for "their inefficiency in handling the case before the drug court". The judge said the prosecution had failed to demonstrate the charges due to the inability and inefficiency of the case investigation officer. Of the five officials, only Mizanur Rahman and his wife Sheuli were present during the delivery of the verdict. The rest of the accused persons are still absconding. The public prosecutor of this case, Dr. Nadim Miah, expressed his disappointment over the verdict by saying to the Dhaka Tribune: "We will decide on moving against the verdict after receiving the copy of the full verdict" [27]. Five prosecution witnesses gave depositions before the court during the trial, sources said. Twenty-eight children across Bangladesh died from renal failure during the period between June and August 2009, after consuming a paracetamol syrup manufactured by Rid Pharma. As the number of deaths was spread around the population, the government published notices in national daily newspapers warning people to not consume any drugs manufactured by this pharma company. A case was filed on August 10th, 2009, by the drug superintendent Shafiqul Islam with the Dhaka drug court against the five accused. Four more petitions were signed in Brahmanbaria, Comilla, Narayanganj and Sylhet. On July 22nd, 2009, the Directorate General of Drug Administration took steps to seal off the Rid Pharma's factory at Brahmanbaria. The national government also constituted a seven-member enquiry committee to probe the matter. On July 29th, 2009, the enquiry committee submitted its report, referring that a poisonous chemical named diethylene glycol was used to manufacture the paracetamol syrup. The report also said that Rid Pharma used diethylene glycol, mainly applied in tannery and rubber industries, as a cheaper substitute of propylene glycol, since diethylene glycol costed Tk. 200 per liter, while propylene glycol costed Tk. 1,100 [26–29].

4. WHO's program on global patient safety challenge (also known as well-being program)

The WHO has the responsibility to promote the health and hygiene of the people of its member countries. To perform this responsibility, WHO has taken a few programs. One of such programs is the Global Patient Safety Challenge. Till date, WHO has undertaken three Global Patient Safety Challenges, which are popularly known as '**Well-being Programs**'. These include [30]:

i. First Global Patient Safety Challenge: **Wash your Hands**

ii. Second Global Patient Safety Challenge: **Safe Surgery** and

iii. 3rd Global Patient Safety/Security Challenge: **Medication without Harm**

These programs are almost self-explanatory, and a detailed description is out of the scope of this chapter.

5. Pharmacovigilance (PV)

According to WHO, PV can be defined as: "the science and activities relating to the detection, assessment, understanding and prevention of adverse effects or any other drug-related problem" [31]. The term PV has been accrued from the Greek word *Pharmakon* meaning *drug* and from the Latin term *vigilare* meaning *to keep aware or, vigilant/alert or, to keep watch* [31]. Vigilance usually indicates:

- Aware/Alert;
- Restraint/Forbearance of sleep, wakefulness;
- Watchfulness in respect of jeopardy, care, caution;
- The procedure of giving close and continuous attention.

From the definition given above, we see that there are four pillars of PV. These include:

i. Detection

ii. Assessment

iii. Understanding (Analysis) and

iv. Prevention (Reporting) of ADR

5.1 Main aims

The general aims of PV are to promote both patient care and patient safety with respect to the use of drugs and medical devices; and to bolster the public health programs (PHP) by giving reliable and equalized information for the productive estimation of the benefit–risk quotient of medicines [32].

The most important aims and purposes of PV are [32];

i. to alert people, not to scare them;

ii. to boost the care and safety of the patient with respect to the consumption of medicines, medical devices and other healthcare interventions;

iii. to improve the public health and safety, while using medicines;

iv. to detect problems of medicine usage, reduce risks and communicate the observations in a disciplined way;

v. to contribute to the evaluation of benefit, hazard, effectiveness and dangers of medicines, directing to the curbing of harm and maximization of beneficial effects;

vi. to embolden the safe, effective (i.e., cost-effective) and rational applications of medicines;

vii. to enhance the understanding, education and the scientific and clinical tutelage in PV and its fruitful communication to the people.

6. PV analytical tools

It is well-known that PV is a risk management procedure for drugs. The process begins with identification of a possible danger, which is then assessed and investigated, ultimately resulting in actions that are taken to minimize those risks. The PV implementation requires the use of specific tools (**Figures 5** and **6**) that will help to communicate with the prescribers and end-users, and the last step should be an evaluation of the effectiveness of the process. The overall process of risk management is iterative due to new proofs that may emerge, or to certain measures taken that may be inadequate. A drug safety issue is rarely considered complete and the safety study goes on until the life cycle completion of the drug.

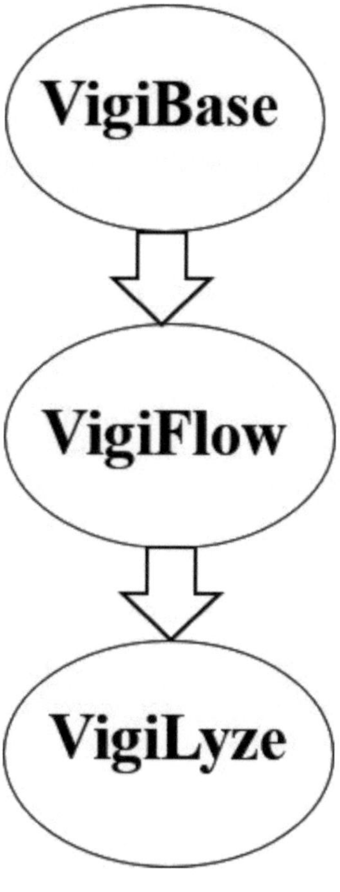

Figure 5.
PV tools to detect and assess the signals related to ADRs.

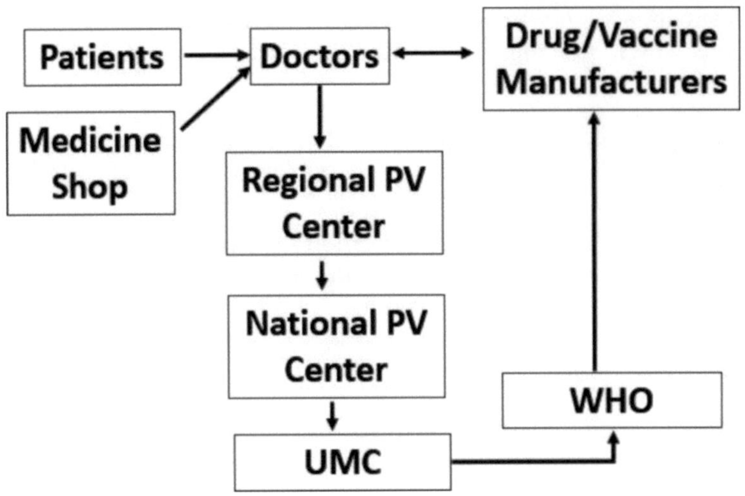

Figure 6.
Flow of information among PV centers and the global monitoring organizations by using PV analytical tools for ADRs analysis [33].

The beginning of the process is normally a 'signal' which is not often a real hazard. Before that can occur, there is a necessity to detect the signal.

The term 'signal' is defined by WHO as a "reported information on a possible causal relationship between an adverse event and a drug, the relationship being unknown or incompletely recorded previously" [34].

6.1 VigiBase

VigiBase is the starting point for the journey of Uppsala Monitoring Center (UMC) from data to wisdom regarding the safe use of drugs, as well as the sage therapeutic decisions in clinical practice. This is the motivating-force of the work of UMC and the WHO Program. The main aim of VigiBase is to make sure that initial signs of previously undetected, unknown, and unexplored drug-related safety problems are identified as quickly as possible.

VigiBase is one of the unique WHO global databases of individual case safety reports (ICSRs). This is the biggest database of its kind worldwide, with more than 20 million reported records of suspected adverse effects of drugs, which have been submitted since 1968 by member states of the WHO PIDM. VigiBase is continually updated with incoming reports from the member countries [35].

6.2 VigiFlow

VigiFlow stands as a management procedure for recording, processing, and sharing reports of ADRs. VigiFlow collects the domestic data and processes the ICSR, thus sharing the reports for instance with VigiBase. This allows maximum local control and gives effective ways for management review and data scanning coming from national sources [36].

6.3 VigiLyze

VigiLyze is a signal detection and management system using national, regional or global data as the launching point for quantitative signal detection. VigiLyze supports the overall signal management process, including the qualitative evaluation.

The major strengths of this signal detection tool are its capacity to re-estimate disproportionality based on any selected country or region background within seconds, and re-investigate those for certainty using different tools [37]. VigiLyze will enable the users to search for any drug or reaction that is shared with the program from UMC, other national centers, or their own centers.

VigiLyze is accessible free of cost to national pharmacovigilance centers in all member states of the WHO Program for IDM. Under-reporting is a familiar matter in pharmacovigilance. By distributing the national reports of adverse events to the global database, individual nations can help increase all countries' understanding of achievable safety concerns.

VigiLyze provides a national, regional, and global aspects of the suspected adverse effects of a drug. This enormous collection of data enhances assessments of surfacing domestic issues. Through VigiLyze it is possible to obtain easy entrance to post-marketing safety information for medicines that are new to the national market, but that are already marketed in other parts of the globe [38].

It is important to mention that one of the major concerns of PV is the safety issue of the PHP [39], such as vaccination in the form of national immunization day, administration of anthelmintics, administration of vitamin A capsule, etc. In those cases, PV tools act as very essential weapons to analyze the situations or adverse effects arising from mass drug administration [40] to handle the pandemics.

7. Bangladesh perspective of PV activities

The Directorate General of Drug Administration (DGDA), under the ministry of Health and Family Welfare, is the national DRA of Bangladesh. The DGDA acts as the only PV center in Bangladesh. An Adverse Drug Reaction Monitoring (ADRM) cell has been set up under the DGDA in 1999 in Bangladesh [41]. The ADR reporting form was introduced in relevant medical institutions to collect information on ADRs. More recently, and under the ADRM, a PV cell was established to effectively monitor and collect the information on ADRs. However, PV is only one of the main components of effective medicine regulation by the national drug regulatory agencies. The vision of DGDA is to guarantee that effective, high-quality and safe drugs are available to the Bangladesh population. This can be achieved through

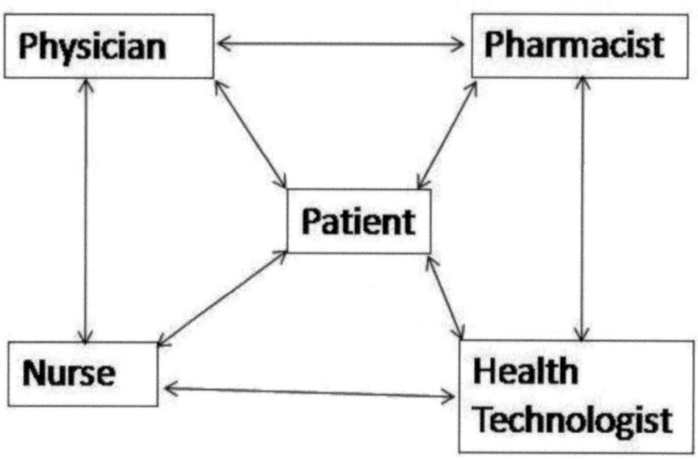

Figure 7.
Interrelationship among the different health professionals (physicians, pharmacists, nurses and health technologists) and the patients [42].

an effective dissemination of the PV cell activities all over the country, including all public and private medical institutes, hospitals, clinics, public and private practitioners, pharmacists, nurses, and other health professionals (**Figure 7**). However, it is very important to keep in mind that the patients should always remain at the center of all [41].

8. Conclusions

The main purpose of the PV study is to protect the future generations or the potential users from the harmful effects of a drug that has already launched in the market. Although the emergence of side effects resulting from the use of drugs are unavoidable, the incidence of morbidity and mortality caused by the occurrence of side effects can be reduced if proper measures are promptly adopted by the local, as well as by the global regulatory organizations. To this end, the main PV principles should be strictly followed by all the member countries of the WHO.

Acknowledgements

1. Dr. Md. Aktar Hossain, Assistant Director, Directorate General of Drug Administration (DGDA).

2. Mr. Ahmed Kamrul Alam, Director (Marketing), Square Pharmaceutical Industry Ltd., Dhaka, Bangladesh.

3. Ariful Karim, Department of Pharmacy, Southeast University, Dhaka, Bangladesh.

Conflict of interest

The author declares no conflict of interest.

Notes/Thanks/Other declarations

Special thank goes to my wife Shirotaz Begum for her cooperation to complete this write up.

Appendices and nomenclature

ADR	Adverse Drug Reaction
ADRM	Adverse Drug Reaction Monitoring
BMJ	British Medical Journal
DGDA	Directorate General of Drug Administration
DRA	Drug Regulatory Authorities
FDA	Food and Drug Administration
ICSR	Individual Case Safety Reports
IDM	International Drug Monitoring
GPSC	Global Patient Safety Challenge
PHP	Public Health Programs

DOI: http://dx.doi.org/10.5772/intechopen.98583

PIDM	Program for International Drug Monitoring
PV	Pharmacovigilance
UMC	Uppsala Monitoring Center
WHO	World Health Organization

Author details

Md. Shah Amran
Department of Pharmaceutical Chemistry, Faculty of Pharmacy, University of Dhaka, Shahbag, Dhaka, Bangladesh

*Address all correspondence to: amranms@du.ac.bd

References

[1] Summarized narratives of Dr. Md. Shah Amran from his experience gained in specialized training on Pharmacovigilance [Specialized training on Pharmacovigilance, Delhi, India, March 03-15, 2019].

[2] Chung Chow Chan, Y C Lee, Herman Lam, Xue-Ming Zhang; Analytical method validation and Instrument performance verification, WILEY-INTERSCIENCE, 2004, 2p.

[3] Guideline for Good Clinical Practice. International Conference on Harmonization of Technical Requirements for Registration of Pharmaceuticals for Human Use. 10 June 1996. 2p.

[4] Nebeker JR, Barach P, Samore MH; Clarifying adverse drug events: a clinician's guide to terminology, documentation, and reporting. Annals of Internal Medicine, 2004. 140 (10): 795-801.

[5] https://www.who.int/teams/regulation-prequalification/pharmacovigilance (Accessed on 15-01-2021)

[6] Neil Vargesson, Thalidomide-Induced Teratogenesis: History and Mechanisms, Birth Defects Research (Part C), 2015, 105:140-156.

[7] WHO Collaborating Centre for International Drug Monitoring, https://www.who.int/medicines/areas/quality_safety/safety_efficacy/collab-centre-uppsala/en/ (Accessed on 15-01-2021)

[8] Members of the WHO Programme for International Drug Monitoring, Full and associate member countries of the WHO Programme and the year they joined. Full member countries (143), https://www.who-umc.org/global-pharmacovigilance/who-programme-for-international-drug-monitoring/who-programme-members/ (Accessed on 15-01-2021)

[9] Bangladesh National Formulary (BDNF), 2015, Volume 4, Pp759-768.

[10] Rashmi R. Shah, Importance of Publishing Adverse Drug Reaction Case Reports: Promoting Public Health and Advancing Pharmacology and Therapeutics, Drug Saf - Case Rep., 2017, 4:11 doi:10.1007/s40800-017-0053-0.

[11] Chung Chow Chan, Herman Lam, Y. C. Lee, Xue-Ming Zhang, Analytical method validation and instrument performance verification, Wiley interscience, 2004, P1-11.

[12] https://penlighten.com/meaning-origin-of-idiom-tip-of-iceberg (accessed on 15-01-2021)

[13] W.G. McBride, THALIDOMIDE AND CONGENITAL ABNORMALITIES, The Lancet, 1961, Volume 278, Issue 7216, 1358p.

[14] Papers of William McBride, ca. 1953-1996, National Library of Australia, accessed 26 July 2010.

[15] Bara Fintel, Athena T. Samaras, Edson Carias, The Thalidomide Tragedy: Lessons for drug safety and regulation, Helix Magazine, Jul 28, 2009.

[16] Attacking the devil: the thalidomide story, BMJ 2016; 352 [BMJ 2016;352:i353]

[17] Md. Shah Amran and Md. Aktar Hossain, Pharmacovigilance and Bangladesh perspective, Bangla Academy Science Journal, 2019, 1:88-95.

[18] "Time Magazine" Archived 3 September 2009 at the Wayback Machine.

[19] Medical Tribunal of New South Wales Archived 20 September 2009 at the Wayback Machine.

[20] Dr. McBride hails end of the affair – "The Australian".

[21] Carol Ballentine, Sulfanilamide Disaster, FDA Consumer magazine, June 1981 Issue.

[22] West, Nancy. "History of Tylenol" (PDF). Nancy West Communications. Retrieved July 26, 2014.

[23] Dan Fletcher, A Brief History of the Tylenol Poisonings, The Time, Monday, Feb 09, 2009.

[24] Euromonitor International. "Acetaminophen benefits from concerns surrounding safety of analgesics". Market Research World. Retrieved July 26, 2014.

[25] Hanif, M., Mobarak, M.R., Ronan, A., Rahman, D., Donovan, J.J. and Bennish, M.L. 1995. Fatal renal failure caused by diethylene glycol in paracetamol elixir: the Bangladesh epidemic. Bri. Med. J.311, 88-91.

[26] The Daily Star, Three Adflame officials jailed for 10yrs, 03:56 PM, July 22, 2014 / LAST MODIFIED: 01:53 AM, March 08, 2015.

[27] The Dhaka Tribune, All acquitted in Rid Pharma paracetamol case, 12:25 pm November 28th, 2016.

[28] The Daily Star, Rid's syrup unauthorized, toxic element found, 11:00 PM, July 29, 2009 / LAST MODIFIED: 11:00 PM, July 29, 2009.

[29] The Daily Star, The unfortunate case of Rid Pharma, 12:00 AM, December 06, 2016 / LAST MODIFIED: 12:00 AM, December 06, 2016.

[30] https://www.who.int/patientsafety/events/05/GPSC_Launch_ENGLISH_FINAL.pdf (Accessed on 01-12-2020)

[31] WHO / Pharmacovigilance (Accessed on 01-12-2020).

[32] WHO / Pharmacovigilance (Accessed on 16-06-2019).

[33] Maria Delaney, Improving pharmacovigilance through direct patient reporting, Cancerworld, March / April 2017. 77:28-32.

[34] https://www.who-umc.org/media/164092/general-information-about-signal-published-in-who-pn.pdf (21-05-2021)

[35] https://www.who-umc.org/vigibase/vigibase/

[36] https://www.who-umc.org/global-pharmacovigilance/vigiflow/

[37] WHOcausality_assessment.pdf (21-05-2021)

[38] https://www.who-umc.org/vigibase/vigilyze/

[39] The SAFETY of MEDICINES IN PUBLIC HEALTH PROGRAMMES: Pharmacovigilance an essential tool, 2006, Pp 9.

[40] https://en.wikipedia.org/wiki/Mass_drug_administration (Accessed on 17-01-2021)

[41] https://www.dgda.gov.bd/index.php/2013-03-31-04-35-57/adrm-news (21-05-2021)

[42] Md. Shah Amran, Introduction to Pharmacy, Published by Krishnachura Publications, Central Road, Dhaka-1205, Dhaka, Bangladesh, 2nd edition, 2015, Pp-7.

Chapter 3

Adverse Drug Reactions Associated with Anti-Tuberculosis Therapy

Vivekanandan Kalaiselvan, Shatrunajay Shukla, Santhanakrishnan Ramesh Kumar, Nikita Mishra, Pawan Kumar and Rajeev Singh Raghuvanshi

Abstract

The pharmacovigilance has been evolved as a professional and ethical practice in ensuring the safety of medicines. The Adverse Drug Reactions (ADRs) associated with the use of medicines including Anti-Tuberculous Therapy (ATT) through a robust system of pharmacovigilance helps in promoting the safety of patients at large. The occurrence of ADRs associated with the use of ATT is expected, a large number of medicines are combined and used for prolonged duration. The suspected ADRs associated with first line ATT are well documented. However, the drugs used in second line or multidrug resistant to tuberculosis (TB), namely bedaquiline, reported to cause QT prolongation in electrocardiogram reading as one of the most common ADRs. Therefore, early identification and prevention of ADRs during ATT is essential for promoting the rational use and reduce the burden of anti-microbial resistance, besides achieving better treatment outcomes.

Keywords: Adverse Drug Reactions, Anti-Tuberculosis Therapy, Bedaquiline, Pharmacovigilance

1. Introduction

The unfortunate tragedy of thalidomide, in 1962, triggered the emergence and implementation of pharmacovigilance across the globe [1]. Thalidomide was introduced in Germany in 1957 and was widely prescribed for the treatment of morning sickness and nausea in pregnant women. Later it was found that babies were born with shortened or absence of limbs (medically known as phocomelia). In 1962, thalidomide was discontinued from the market due to the increased number of scientific reports describing numerous cases of phocomelia [2]. This tragedy led to the creation of the World Health Organization (WHO) pilot research project for International Drug Monitoring in 1968, with the purpose to develop a system and tools applicable internationally, for detecting previously unknown or poorly understood adverse drug reactions (ADRs) of medicines [3]. Currently, this network has been expanded to more than 140 developed, low- and middle-income countries. These 140 countries participated in the WHO programme for international drug monitoring as member states, and 31 countries have also joined as associate member states. These countries have established pharmacovigilance system at their capacity, to monitor the medication safety. WHO and its collaborating centres are continuously providing technical support for capacity building and strengthening of these pharmacovigilance systems [4].

As per WHO, Pharmacovigilance is defined as a "science of detection, assessment, understanding and prevention of ADRs or any other drug related problems" [5]. This enables the scope of clinical practice of monitoring & reporting of ADRs, analyses the information and sharing the learnings with healthcare providers for prevention of such ADRs, for better patient's safety and outcomes. Pharmacovigilance and its concepts are evolving as one of the most important components in contemporary clinical and regulatory practice. In clinical trials, most medicines will only be tested for short-term safety and efficacy on a limited number of carefully selected individuals (excluding pregnant women, children and elderly). In some cases, as few as 500, and rarely more than 5000, subjects receive the investigational new drug prior to its release [6]. It is not possible to identify and record many ADRs in such a shorter duration, protected environment and restricted population in trials. After stage three of clinical trial, the medicine is available to be launch in the market and is legally set free for consumption by the general population. Post market experience has shown that many adverse effects, interactions (i.e. with foods or other medicines), and risk factors may come to light even after several years of introducing the medicine into the market [7]. Moreover, many studies have shown that an ADR may result into a significantly decrease in the quality of life, increased hospitalizations, prolonged hospital stay and mortality [8]. Therefore, monitoring the safety of the medicines throughout its life period is pivotal, as most of the ADRs are usually reported during prolonged use.

The pharmacovigilance practice applies equally to medicines used in public health programs, including medicines used in Anti-Tubercular Therapy (ATT). As the management of tuberculosis (TB) involves longer duration of therapy and also multiple drugs, these arise as predisposing factors for the occurrence of ADRs [9]. Such ADRs pose a challenge in the management of TB. Though it is a prolonged treatment, medication must be continued in order to ensure the compliance, otherwise it will end with treatment failure or developing antimicrobial resistance [10]. Generally, patients discontinue the medication due to the emergence of ADRs resulting from the administration of first-line anti-TB drugs. During the course of TB treatment, there may be a risk of morbidity and mortality, particularly with drug-induced hepatitis. Therefore, there are public health program in various countries that systematically monitor, prevent and manage ADRs encountered during the treatment of TB, in order to achieve maximum treatment outcomes [11].

TB is a chronic infection caused primarily by *Mycobacterium tuberculosis*. The lung is generally the first affected organ, as the infection is usually due to inhalation of infected droplet nuclei. Approximately 80% of the TB cases are pulmonary TB [12]. Around 30% patients who are infected with Human Immune Deficiency Virus (HIV) will also develop active tuberculosis. Factors, such as HIV, Resistant TB, drug–drug interactions raise the complexity of problem. As per the WHO strategy, directly observed treatment short-course (DOTS) therapy for the duration of 6–8 months is one of the important components for the treatment of TB. The short-course therapy is usually performed in 2 phases: the initial phase (2 months) involves the concurrent use of at least 3 drugs to rapidly reduce the bacterial population and prevent emergence of drug-resistant bacteria. The second, continuation phase, (4–6 months) involves fewer drugs and is used to eliminate any remaining bacteria and prevent recurrence. Worldwide, HIV infection has been identified as an important predisposing factor of immune-suppression leading to TB [13]. It increases the susceptibility to primary infection and increases the reactivation rate

First line drugs given for Drug Sensitive TB	New patients with pulmonary TB should receive a regimen containing 6 months of rifampicin: (Isoniazid + Rifampicin + Pyrazinamide + Ethambutol) *In populations with known or suspected high levels of isoniazid resistance, new TB patients may receive HRE as therapy in the continuation phase. Recommended: 1. Daily dosage 2. Fixed Dose Combination drugs
Second line drugs given for Rifampicin Resistance/Multi Drug Resistance/Extremely Druf Resistance (RR/MDR/XDR) TB and Multi Drug Resistance (MDR-TB)	Group A: Fluoroquinolones Levofloxacin, Moxifloxacin, Gatifloxacin
	Group B: Second-line injectable agents Amikacin, Capreomycin, Kanamycin, (Streptomycin)
	Group C: Other core second-line agents Ethionamide/prothionamide, Cycloserine/terizidone, Linezolid, Clofazimine
	Group D: Add-on agents (not part of the core MDR-TB regimen), D1 Pyrazinamide Ethambutol,High-dose isoniazid
	D2 Bedaquiline,Delamanid
	D3 p-aminosalicylic acid, Imipenem–cilastatind Meropenem, Amoxicillin-clavulanated (Thioacetazone)

Table 1.
Recommended drugs used to treat tuberculosis.

of TB [14]. Although this regimen is effective in treating active TB, it is associated with many ADRs and poses a significant challenge to completion of treatment. Recommended treatment regimens for TB are given in **Table 1**.

2. Importance of ADR reporting in tuberculosis

Multiple types of drug therapy are given for TB, and even new TB patients (sensitive to first-line drugs), are receiving a treatment regimen with a combination of four drugs [15]. There is a chance for developing ADR either for one or the combination of drugs, and that has to be identified for ensuring a sustained treatment compliance, till the completion of ATT. When treatment is given to patients with TB-associated drug resistance, either ionized resistance, multidrug resistance or rifampicin resistance, pre-extensively drug resistance or extensively drug resistance TB, the number of drugs given could be higher, and it becomes imperative to identify the resulting/associated ADRs. In case any ADR takes place, the treatment management has to be done appropriately [16]. For TB patients having HIV co-infection, the treatment given for HIV infection, including the antiretroviral therapy, and/or the medication given for the associated conditions, may overlap with the ADR presented, and so it becomes very important to monitor this group of population for efficient management. In addition, also in TB patients with special medical conditions associated, like associated diabetes mellitus, liver, renal or seizure disorders, and psychosis, the treatment should be done cautiously, by closely observing the progress and monitoring all the ADRs encountered. Furthermore, when new drugs like Bedaquiline (BDQ), Delamanid (DLM) and Pretomanid are initiated at TB programs, it is essential that the associated ADRs are captured promptly for effective management of TB [17].

2.1 ADRs associated with first-line anti-TB drugs

The ATT is expected to cause more ADRs, because it involves combination of several medicines and is used for a longer duration [9]. One of the most common ADRs observed with the administration of ATT is gastrointestinal symptoms, such as nausea, vomiting etc. These ADRs could be symptomatically managed without the need for a change in the dosage of drugs. The hepatotoxicity is also a risk associated with ATT, and its frequency can range from 2–39% in different countries [18]. As compared to Western population, Indian sub-population studies reported high incidence of hepatotoxicity with ATT [19].

2.1.1 Isoniazid

Isoniazid has been shown to be well tolerated at recommended dose. However, systemic or cutaneous hypersensitivity reactions can occasionally occur during the first weeks of treatment [15]. By daily supplementary dose of pyridoxine in vulnerable patients, the risk of peripheral neuropathy can be excluded. In the later stages of treatement, some susceptible patients can develop neurological disturbance, encompassing optic neuritis, toxic psychosis and generalized convulsions. This may require the discontinuation of isoniazid. An uncommon but potentially serious reaction is symptomatic hepatitis, which could be precluded by prompt withdrawal of treatment. Asymptomatic rise in serum concentrations of hepatic transaminases at the beginning of treatment has very low clinical significance. The same resolves spontaneously as the treatment carry on. Other rare adverse effects linked with isoniazid are lupus-like syndrome, pellagra, anemia, and arthralgias [20].

2.1.2 Rifampicin

At currently recommended doses, this drug has been shown to be well tolerated by most of the patients. Occasionally it may cause gastrointestinal reactions including abdominal pain, nausea, vomiting and pruritus with or without rash [21]. With an intermittent drug administration, adverse effects, such as fever, influenza-like syndrome and thrombocytopenia may occur. In HIV-positive TB patients, exfoliative dermatitis is more common. Patients taking the drug 3 times a week, adverse effects including temporary oliguria, dyspnoea and haemolytic anemia have been reported. If the regimen is changed to daily dosage these reactions usually subsided. In the beginning of treatment, moderate rises in serum concentrations of bilirubin and transaminases are common adverse effects are often transient and not clinical significant. A potentially fatal condition is dose-related hepatitis, it is therefore important to not exceed the maximum recommended daily dose of 600 mg.

2.1.3 Pyrazinamide

This drug has been reported to cause various skin reactions, like maculopapular rash, erythema multiforme, exfoliative dermatitis and drug rash with eosinophilia and systemic symptoms (DRESS) syndrome. Among the first-line drugs, pyrazinamide has shown to be the most common drug to cause cutaneous ADRs [22]. Pyrazinamide may cause gastrointestinal intolerance. Hypersensitivity reactions are rare, but have been reported in some patients with modest flushed skin. During the early phases of the treatment, moderate rises in serum transaminase concentrations are common. A rare complication is severe hepatotoxicity. A degree of hyperuricaemia may also occur asymptomatically as a result of inhibition of renal tubular secretion [15]. The treatment may also result into gout, which can be treated with allopurinol. Arthralgia, especially of the shoulders, may occur which can be treated with simple analgesics (especially aspirin). By prescribing regimens with intermittent administration of pyrazinamide, hyperuricaemia and arthralgia may be eliminated. Sideroblastic anemia and photosensitive dermatitis are some of the rare ADRs associated with this drug [7, 8].

2.1.4 Streptomycin

Streptomycin injections are painful, and rash, induration, or sterile abscesses can be formed at injection sites. Numbness and tingling around the mouth occur immediately after injection and cutaneous hypersensitivity reactions can occur. The incidence of ototoxicity associated with the use of ATT may be as high as 25% [23]. With currently recommended doses, the complications like impairment of vestibular function are uncommon. Vertigo is more common than hearing loss. Indications of injury at the 8th cranial (auditory) nerve include ringing in the ears, ataxia, vertigo and deafness. The damage is impermanent and can be reversed by reducing in dosage, or the stopping the treatment with this drug. This damage is commonly occurs within the first 2 months of treatment. More commonly, the other aminoglycoside antibiotics e.g. kanamycin, amikacin and capreomycin are more nephrotoxic than streptomycin. If urinary output falls, albuminuria occurs, or tubular casts are detected in the urine, streptomycin should be stopped, and renal function should be evaluated.

Though WHO's recommendation is not to use injectable streptomycin, we should take into consideration that other recommended treatments with aminoglycosides may cause similar types of ADRs [17].

2.1.5 Ethambutol

Dose-dependent optic neuritis caused by Ethambutol can result in impairment of visual acuity and color vision in one or both eyes. Early changes are usually reversible, but blindness can occur if treatment is not discontinued promptly. Ocular toxicity is rare when ethambutol is used for 2–3 months at recommended doses. Peripheral neuropathy has been reported in approximately 20% of patients treated with ethambutol. Other rare adverse events include generalized cutaneous reaction, arthralgia and, very rarely, hepatitis [24].

Several studies have reported that the drugs used to treat TB may cause ADRs. Management and prevention of such ADRs are important measures to be adopted to increase tolerance. Generally, with non-serious ADRs, the drugs do not need to be stopped, while with serious ADRs, the drugs often have to be stopped and a modified regimen has to be implemented [9].

2.1.6 Capreomycin

This drug is administered in combination with other first-line drugs. The common ADRs reported are hypersensitivity reactions, including urticaria and rashes, nephrotoxicity, electrolyte disturbance, hearing loss wit tinnitus and vertigo [11].

Grading of toxicity associated with drugs used for TB treatment and the ADRs associated with the anti-TB drugs used for therapy are given in **Tables 2** and **3**, respectively.

Grade & Level	Toxicity
1 - Mild	Transient or mild discomfort; no limitation in activity; no medical intervention or therapy required.
2 – Moderate	Mild to moderate limitation in activity, some assistance may be needed; none or minimal medical intervention or therapy required.
3 - Severe	Marked limitation in activity, some assistance usually required; medical intervention or therapy required, hospitalization is possible.
4 – Life threatening	Extreme limitation in activity, significant assistance required; significant medical intervention or therapy required, hospitalization or hospice care are probable.

Table 2.
Grades of toxicity resulting from TB treatment [25].

Adverse Drug Reaction	Symptoms and signs	Responsible Drug
Audiovestibular manifestations	Hearing loss, vertigo, new-onset tinnitus	Aminoglycosides, Capreomycin
Blood sugar abnormalities	Dizziness, sweating, fainting, poor response to infections	Fluorquinolones (FQ), Rifampicin (R), Pyrazinamide (Z)
Dermatitis	Itching, rash, hives, fever, petechial rash	Pyrazinamide, Rifampicin, Thiacetazone
Gastro-intestinal	Anorexia, nausea, vomiting, epigastric pain	Pyrazinamide, Rifampicin; p-Aminosalicylic acid
Hematology	Leucopenia, thrombocytopenia, anemia, eosinophilia	Rifampicin (intermittent); Linezolid, Isoniazid, capreomycin
Hepatitis	Anorexia, nausea, vomiting, jaundice, abdominal pain	Isoniazid, Rifampicin, Ethambutol, Pyrazinamide
Hypothyroidism	Fatigue, weight gain, depression	P-aminosalicylic acid, pro/ Etionamide
Joint, tendon	Gout-like manifestations; SLE; tendinopathies	Pyrazinamide; Isoniazid (Rarelyrifampicin); Fluorquinolones;
Neuro/psychiatric	Headaches, depression, agitation; suicidal ideation	Isoniazid, Fluorquinolones, Cycloserine
Peripheral neuropathy	Numb feet or hands	Ionizedlinezolid; Cycloserine, Aminoglycosides
Renal impairment	Uraemia; haematuria	Aminoglycosides, Capreomycin; Rifampicin (intermittent)
Visual disorders	Vision loss and color blindness; uveitis	Ethambutol, Linezolid; Rifabutin, Rifapentane;

Table 3.
Most common ADRs associated with the use of anti-TB drugs.

2.2 ADRs associated with second-line anti-TB drugs

Resistant -TB is usually treated with a combination of drugs that are more toxic than isoniazid and rifampicin. These drugs include fluoroquinolones, aminoglycosides, ethionamide, cycloserine, aminosalicyclic acid, linezolid and clofazimine, among others [26]. The main ADRs associated with the use of cycloserine are reported as neurological disorders, including headache, dizziness, vertigo, drowsiness, tremor, convulsions, confusion, psychosis, depression, rashes, allergic dermatitis, megaloblastic anemia, and changes in liver function tests [27]. Minor adverse effects are relatively common, and they can be easily managed with symptomatic treatment. However, some adverse effects can be life-threatening, for example, nephrotoxicity due to aminoglycosides, cardiotoxicity due to fluoroquinolones, gastrointestinal toxicity due to ethionamide or para-amino-salicylic acid, central nervous system toxicity due to cycloserine, etc. [17].

2.3 Multi Drug-resistant TB (MDR-TB)

MDR-TB is caused by organisms that are resistant to isoniazid and rifampicin. As per the WHO reports, an estimated 480 000 worldwide patients developed MDR-TB in 2015, in addition to the 100 000 patients with rifampicin-resistant TB that were newly eligible for MDT-TB treatment [22]. Again, according to WHO, the second highest MDR-TB incident country in the world, China, accounted for 45% of the 580 000 cases, together with Indian and the Russian Federations, with 6.6% of new TB cases and 30% of previously treated cases having MDR/Rifampicin resistant TB.

The novel anti tubercular drugs, namely BDQ and DLM, now included in WHO second-line treatment [28], as well as in some countries, have received conditional approval for use in adults with MDR-TB. BDQ, a new anti TB- drug, has been given approval by the United States Food and Drug Administration in 2012 [29], and by the European Medicines Agency in 2014. In India, BDQ was introduced under the conditional access program in 2015. The safety profile and tolerability of a BDQ-containing treatment regimen used in India has been established. QT prolongation in electrocardiogram reading has been reported as one of the most common ADRs with the use of BDQ; the others include peripheral neuropathy, vomiting, breathlessness and thrombocytopenia [30].

2.4 Prevalence of adverse events associated with second-line anti-TB drugs in children

Children, especially those under 10 years old, can tolerate second-line combination of anti-TB drugs better than adults. In children, the higher rate of ADRs has been observed in those having HIV as comorbid infection, as compared to TB infection alone [14]. Several studies have also revealed that the majority of the adverse events found in children are mild to moderate, thus not requiring interruption or complete cessation of treatment. Moreover, even with the occurrence of few severe adverse events, permanent discontinuation of drugs is rarely necessary [14].

The second–line drugs are generally found to cause more ADRs, as compared to the first-line drugs [31]. The healthcare workers treating children should be aware of this fact and should thus be able to manage such ADRs. Healthcare workers, care givers or parents are required to be trained accordingly, because most of the children may not be able to report the drug-associated ADRs. The MDR-TB treatment outcomes in children are well achieved in many countries by using the currently available drugs [32, 33]. However, the improvement of the MDR-TB treatment programme can be achieved by: (1) implementing targeted or cohort event monitoring of adverse events, with the use of MDR-TB drugs in children; and (2) healthcare works training for a timely ADRs reporting, aiming to achieve the maximum treatment outcomes.

2.5 Causality and severity assessment of anti-TB drugs-associated adverse events

After determining the adverse events (suspected) of anti-TB drugs, the very next step is to establish the causal or temporal relationship between the drug and the event, i.e., is the drug actually causing the event? It is possible that the administered drug and the occurrence of an adverse event may have a close temporal relationship, but still not be a reaction [34].

Having considered the parameters in assessing the temporal relationship, the next step is to address the following question: "Did these medicines actually cause the event?" In other words, "Is the event a reaction?" It is conceivable/acceptable that the administration of a medicine and the occurrence of an event may have a close relationship, but still not be a reaction, for example, death from myocardial infarction. In actual practice, the assessment of the relationship and causality frequently merge, particularly when an event is a well-known reaction and the relationship is close. The two phases occur without conscious deliberation, but should be there nevertheless. However, it is often necessary to gather other knowledge about the medicine, the patient and the event, in order to undertake a deliberate evaluation of these factors, which are actually external to the drug–event association that has occurred. Causality assessment is the methodological approach for evaluating a signal (identification of new safety alert) [35]. As per WHO, the causality assessment scale is the estimated strength of the relationship between the drug and the ADR can be classified as certain, probable, possible, unlikely, conditional/unclassified,

Certain	• Event of laboratory test abnormality, with plausible time relationship to drug intake • Cannot be explained by disease or other drugs • Response to withdrawal plausible (pharmacologically, pathologically) • Event definitive pharmacologically or phenomenological (An objective and specific medical disorders or a recognized pharmacological phenomenon) • Rechallenge (if necessary)
Probable	• Event or lab test abnormality, with reasonable time relationship during intake • Unlikely to be attributed to disease or other drugs • Response to withdrawal clinically reasonable • Rechallenge not necessary
Possible	• Event or laboratory test abnormality, with reasonable time relationship to drug intake • Could also be explained by disease or other drugs • Information on drug withdrawal lacking or unclear
Unlikely	• Event or laboratory test abnormality with a time to drug that makes a relationship improbable (but not impossible) • Diseases or other drugs provide plausible explanations
Conditional/unclassified	• Event or laboratory test abnormality • More data for proper assessment needed • Or additional data under examination
Unassessable/Unclassifiable	• A report suggesting an adverse reaction • Cannot be judged because of insufficient or contradictory information • Report cannot be supplemented or verified

Table 4.
WHO's scale for causality assessment [36].

S. No.	Question	Answer		
		Yes	No	Do Not Know
1	Are there previous conclusive reports on this reaction?	+1	0	0
2	Did the adverse event appear after the suspected drug was administered?	+2	−1	0
3	Did the adverse reaction improve when the drug was discontinued or a specific antagonist was administered?	+1	0	0
4	Did the adverse reaction reappear when the drug was re-administered?	+2	−1	0
5	Are there alternative causes (other than the drug) that could solely have caused the reaction?	−1	+2	0
6	Did the reaction reappear when a placebo was given?	-1	+1	0
7	Was the drug detected in the blood (or other fluids) in a concentration known to be toxic?	+1	0	0
8	Was the reaction more severe when the dose was increased, or less severe when the dose was decreased?	+1	0	0
9	Did the patient have a similar reaction to the same or similar drugs in any previous exposure?	+1	0	0
10	Was the adverse event confirmed by objective evidence?	+1	0	0

The total score calculated from this table defines the category as:
a. Definite (>9).
b. Probable (5 to 8).
c. Possible (1 to 4).
d. Unlikely (< 0).

Table 5.
Naranjo's scale for causality assessment [37].

unassessable/unclassifiable (**Table 4**). The Naranjo scale can also be applied for causality assessment, and is algorithm-based (**Table 5**) [38].

The severity assessment of ADRs can also be categorized in to into seven levels of severity level 1 and 2 are considered less severe or mild, levels 3 and 4 are moderate, and levels 5, 6 and 7 are classified as severe [39]. Severe level of ADRs includes all potentially life threatening ADRs, and the ones causing permanent damage or requiring intensive medical care. Even some other assessment scales classify severe and lethal.

3. Conclusions

The emergence of ADRs continues to remain an important public health issue worldwide, as it is among the ten leading causes of mortality. Early identification and prevention of ADRs during TB treatment will lead to the rational use of medicines and to a reduce burden of antimicrobial resistance. Better adherence within the target population will reassure that monitoring and good communication on risks and benefits provide favorable implications for decisions on medicine procurement. Safety monitoring of medicines is thus a vital and crucial element of any health system. As TB treatment relies on a multi-drug therapy for long duration, the emergence of ADRs is inevitable. Therefore, ADR reporting is essential as it will strengthen the evidence, maximize the benefits and minimize the risks.

Abbreviations

ADRs	Adverse Drug Reactions
ATT	Anti-Tubercular Therapy
BDQ	Bedaquiline
DLM	Delamanid
DOTS	Directly Observed Treatment Short-Course
HIV	Human Immunodeficiency Viruses
MDR-TB	Multid Drug-Resistant Tuberculosis
TB	Tuberculosis
WHO	World Health Organization
DRESS	Drug Rash with Eosinophilia and Systemic Symptoms syndrome

Author details

Vivekanandan Kalaiselvan[1*], Shatrunajay Shukla[1], Santhanakrishnan Ramesh Kumar[2], Nikita Mishra[1], Pawan Kumar[1] and Rajeev Singh Raghuvanshi[1]

1 Indian Pharmacopoeia Commission, Ministry of Health and Family Welfare, Government of India, Ghaziabad, Uttar Pradesh, India

2 ICMR-National Institute for Research in Tuberculosis, Chennai, India

*Address all correspondence to: vivekarts@gmail.com; kalaiselvan.ipc@gov.in

References

[1] N. Vargesson, "Thalidomide Embryopathy: An Enigmatic Challenge," *ISRN Developmental Biology*, Oct. 31, 2013. https://www.hindawi.com/journals/isrn/2013/241016/ (accessed Feb. 24, 2021).

[2] N. Vargesson, "Thalidomide-induced teratogenesis: history and mechanisms," *Birth Defects Res C Embryo Today*, vol. 105, no. 2, pp. 140-156, Jun. 2015, doi: 10.1002/bdrc.21096.

[3] W. H. Organization, *Handbook of resolutions and decisions of the World Health Assembly and the Executive Board*. World Health Organization, 1973.

[4] D. N. Iessa, "Pharmacovigilance: New Challenges for WHO," p. 52.

[5] "Pharmacovigilance - an overview | ScienceDirect Topics." https://www.sciencedirect.com/topics/pharmacology-toxicology-and-pharmaceutical-science/pharmacovigilance (accessed Feb. 24, 2021).

[6] J. A. Berlin, S. C. Glasser, and S. S. Ellenberg, "Adverse Event Detection in Drug Development: Recommendations and Obligations Beyond Phase 3," *Am J Public Health*, vol. 98, no. 8, pp. 1366-1371, Aug. 2008, doi: 10.2105/AJPH.2007.124537.

[7] N. Raj, S. Fernandes, N. R. Charyulu, A. Dubey, R. G. S., and S. Hebbar, "Postmarket surveillance: a review on key aspects and measures on the effective functioning in the context of the United Kingdom and Canada," *Ther Adv Drug Saf*, vol. 10, Jul. 2019, doi: 10.1177/2042098619865413.

[8] R. I. Thomas, D. J. Cameron, and M. C. Fahs, "A Prospective Study of Delirium and Prolonged Hospital Stay: Exploratory Study," *Archives of General Psychiatry*, vol. 45, no. 10, pp. 937-940, Oct. 1988, doi: 10.1001/archpsyc.1988.01800340065009.

[9] "A practical handbook on the pharmacovigilance of medicines used in the treatment of tuberculosis." Accessed: Mar. 17, 2021. [Online]. Available: https://www.who.int/docs/default-source/documents/tuberculosis/a-practical-handbook-on-the-pharmacovigilance-of-medicines-used-in-the-treatment-of-tuberculosis.pdf?sfvrsn=6e5fc0cf_5.

[10] F. Imam *et al.*, "Adverse drug reaction prevalence and mechanisms of action of first-line anti-tubercular drugs," *Saudi Pharmaceutical Journal*, vol. 28, no. 3, pp. 316-324, Mar. 2020, doi: 10.1016/j.jsps.2020.01.011.

[11] "Pivotal role of Pharmacovigilance Programme of India in containment of antimicrobial resistance in India Agrawal V, Shrivastava TP, Adusumilli PK, Vivekanandan K, Thota P, Bhushan S - Perspect Clin Res." https://www.picronline.org/article.asp?issn=2229-3485;year=2019;volume=10;issue=3;spage=140;epage=144;aulast=Agrawal (accessed Mar. 17, 2021).

[12] C. Hoffmann, "Pulmonary tuberculosis in adults," in *Tuberculosis*, Elsevier, 2009, pp. 332-341.

[13] T. T. Todorova, G. Tsankova, and N. L. and T. Kostadinova, "Tuberculosis and HIV — Doubling the Fatality," *Immunopathology and Immuno modulation*, Nov. 2015, doi: 10.5772/61138.

[14] J. Bruchfeld, M. Correia-Neves, and G. Källenius, "Tuberculosis and HIV Coinfection," *Cold Spring Harb Perspect Med*, vol. 5, no. 7, Jul. 2015, doi: 10.1101/cshperspect.a017871.

[15] World Health Organization and Stop TB Initiative (World Health

Organization), Eds., *Treatment of tuberculosis: guidelines*, 4th ed. Geneva: World Health Organization, 2010.

[16] "WHO_HTM_TB_2014.23_eng.pdf." Accessed: Mar. 17, 2021. [Online]. Available: https://apps.who.int/iris/bitstream/handle/10665/137334/WHO_HTM_TB_2014.23_eng.pdf;jsessionid=3F28C9E7FB3CC604788D92E5CEB971F8?sequence=1.

[17] World Health Organization, *WHO consolidated guidelines on drug-resistant tuberculosis treatment.* 2019.

[18] "Risk Factors of Hepatotoxicity During Anti-tuberculosis Treatment." https://www.ncbi.nlm.nih.gov/pmc/articles/PMC4923276/ (accessed Feb. 24, 2021).

[19] P. R *et al.*, "Hepatic toxicity in South Indian patients during treatment of tuberculosis with short-course regimens containing isoniazid, rifampicin and pyrazinamide," *Tubercle*, Jun. 1986. https://pubmed.ncbi.nlm.nih.gov/3775870/ (accessed Feb. 24, 2021).

[20] "WHO | Toman's tuberculosis: case detection, treatment and monitoring: questions and answers (2nd edition)," *WHO*. https://www.who.int/tb/publications/toman/en/ (accessed Feb. 24, 2021).

[21] "Treatment of Tuberculosis American Thoracic Society, CDC, and Infectious Diseases Society of America." https://www.cdc.gov/mmwr/preview/mmwrhtml/rr5211a1.htm (accessed Feb. 24, 2021).

[22] "Prevalence of adverse drug reaction with first-line drugs among patients treated for pulmonary tuberculosis - Clinical Epidemiology and Global Health." https://cegh.net/article/S2213-3984(15)00073–1/fulltext (accessed Feb. 24, 2021).

[23] M. Rd, S. Cr, and L. Ps, "Risk factors for the development of auditory toxicity in patients receiving aminoglycosides," *The Journal of infectious diseases*, Jan. 1984. https://pubmed.ncbi.nlm.nih.gov/6693788/ (accessed Feb. 24, 2021).

[24] X. Lv *et al.*, "Adverse Reactions Due to Directly Observed Treatment Strategy Therapy in Chinese Tuberculosis Patients: A Prospective Study," *PLOS ONE*, vol. 8, no. 6, p. e65037, Jun. 2013, doi: 10.1371/journal.pone.0065037.

[25] C. Sekaggya-Wiltshire *et al.*, "Anti-TB drug concentrations and drug-associated toxicities among TB/HIV-coinfected patients," *J Antimicrob Chemother*, vol. 72, no. 4, pp. 1172-1177, Apr. 2017, doi: 10.1093/jac/dkw534.

[26] K. E. Dooley *et al.*, "Old Drugs, New Purpose: Retooling Existing Drugs for Optimized Treatment of Resistant Tuberculosis," *Clinical Infectious Diseases*, vol. 55, no. 4, pp. 572-581, Aug. 2012, doi: 10.1093/cid/cis487.

[27] "National Formulary of India 5th Edition, 2016, Page 208." Indian Pharmacopoeia Commission.

[28] M. Grzemska, "Updated WHO MDR-TB treatment guidelines and the use of new drugs in children," *Resid Pediatr*, vol. 7, no. Supl, pp. 7-10, Oct. 2017, doi: 10.25060/residpediatr-2017.v7s1-03.

[29] S. Yadav, G. Rawal, and M. Baxi, "Bedaquiline: A Novel Antitubercular Agent for the Treatment of Multidrug-Resistant Tuberculosis," *J Clin Diagn Res*, vol. 10, no. 8, pp. FM01–FM02, Aug. 2016, doi: 10.7860/JCDR/2016/19052.8286.

[30] "Effectiveness and safety of bedaquiline under conditional access program for treatment of drug-resistant tuberculosis in India: An interim analysis - PubMed." https://pubmed.

ncbi.nlm.nih.gov/32192613/ (accessed Feb. 24, 2021).

[31] "First– and Second–Line Drugs and Drug Resistance | IntechOpen." https://www.intechopen.com/books/tuberculosis-current-issues-in-diagnosis-and-management/first-and-second-line-drugs-and-drug-resistance (accessed Feb. 24, 2021).

[32] H. H. Tola, K. J. Khadoura, W. Jimma, S. Nedjat, and R. Majdzadeh, "Multidrug resistant tuberculosis treatment outcome in children in developing and developed countries: A systematic review and meta-analysis," *International Journal of Infectious Diseases*, vol. 96, pp. 12-18, Jul. 2020, doi: 10.1016/j.ijid.2020.03.064.

[33] H. S. Schaaf, S. Thee, L. van der Laan, A. C. Hesseling, and A. J. Garcia-Prats, "Adverse effects of oral second-line antituberculosis drugs in children," *Expert Opin Drug Saf*, vol. 15, no. 10, pp. 1369-1381, Oct. 2016, doi: 10.1080/14740338.2016.1216544.

[34] H. S. Rehan, D. Chopra, and A. K. Kakkar, "Physician's guide to pharmacovigilance: Terminology and causality assessment," *European Journal of Internal Medicine*, vol. 20, no. 1, pp. 3-8, Jan. 2009, doi: 10.1016/j.ejim.2008.04.019.

[35] "UMC | What is a signal?" https://www.who-umc.org/research-scientific-development/signal-detection/what-is-a-signal/ (accessed Mar. 17, 2021).

[36] S. A. Zaki, "Adverse drug reaction and causality assessment scales," *Lung India*, vol. 28, no. 2, pp. 152-153, 2011, doi: 10.4103/0970-2113.80343.

[37] "ADVERSE DRUG REACTION-CAUSALITY ASSESSMENT." Accessed: Mar. 17, 2021. [Online]. Available: http://www.ijrpc.com/files/00050.pdf.

[38] R. P. Naidu, "Causality assessment: A brief insight into practices in pharmaceutical industry," *Perspect Clin Res*, vol. 4, no. 4, pp. 233-236, 2013, doi: 10.4103/2229-3485.120173.

[39] S. C. Hartwig, J. Siegel, and P. J. Schneider, "Preventability and severity assessment in reporting adverse drug reactions," *Am J Hosp Pharm*, vol. 49, no. 9, pp. 2229-2232, Sep. 1992.

Chapter 4

Prevalence and Significance of Antibiotic-Associated Adverse Reactions

Tânia Magalhães Silva, Eva Rebelo Gomes, Inês Ribeiro-Vaz, Fátima Roque and Maria Teresa Herdeiro

Abstract

The World Health Organization (WHO) defines Pharmacovigilance as the science and activities relating to the detection, assessment, understanding and prevention of adverse drug effects. The aim is to promote the safety and effective use of medicines through an early detection and evaluation of drug safety risks. The pharmacovigilance system is essentially based in spontaneous reports of Adverse Drug Reactions (ADR). ADR can be associated with severe outcomes and significant mortality, besides, most of them are deemed to be preventable events. Globally, antibiotics are among the most widely prescribed medications and their extensive use is linked to antibiotic-associated ADR. This chapter aims to summarize available epidemiological data concerning antibiotic use related ADR and analyze the reports received by the EudraVigilance system regarding the exclusive usage of antibiotics.

Keywords: Antibiotics, Adverse Drug Reactions, Pharmacovigilance System

1. Introduction

The history of antibiotics and its use can be dated back to the previous century [1]. According to the World Health Organization (WHO), antibiotics are "medicines used to prevent and treat bacterial infections" [2]. These powerful medicines are used to destroy specific bacteria, or to prevent their spread, thus not being suitable to treat, for instance, viral infections. Over the years, antibiotics have shown to effectively treat several previously life-threatening diseases caused by bacteria, being the first therapeutic approach in those clinical conditions [3, 4].

The appropriate use of antibiotics is safe, effective and has few adverse effects. However, when these medicines are improperly prescribed, bacterial resistance may arise. This problem, commonly known as antibiotic resistance (ABR), is one of the major public health threats of the 21st century worldwide [4, 5]. Globally, the annual predicted number of deaths caused by bacterial agents may increase from 700 thousand million deaths to 10 million by 2050, if no action is adopted [5]. A study based on data from the European Antimicrobial Resistance Surveillance Network (EARS-Net) during 2015 estimated that, annually, around 670 thousand infections occur in the European Union (EU) due to antibiotic-resistant bacteria, with approximately 33 thousand people dying as a direct outcome of these types of infection [6]. The overall crude economic burden of ABR was estimated to be at least 1.5 billion euros a year in the EU, the majority due to hospital costs [7]. Consequently, the fight against ABR stands as an extremely important public health target that should not be underestimated.

The appropriate use of antibiotics is essential to prevent ABR and reduce the risk of adverse reactions. Adverse drug reactions (ADR) are another public health problem, namely in terms of mortality, morbidity and healthcare costs, that requires maximum attention [8]. An ADR can be defined as "a noxious and unintended response to a medicinal product" [9], and can be caused by any drug class. Nevertheless, globally, antibiotics are among the leading drug classes responsible for the occurrence of ADR [10, 11].

Pharmacovigilance systems are essential to enhance patients' care and safety, being responsible for the monitoring of pre-market review and post-market surveillance processes. Moreover, they provide reliable and balanced information for an effective evaluation of the benefits and risks of available medical drugs [12].

The development of educational interventions to improve the awareness of health professionals, and the literacy of the population in general about the dangerous health implications of an inadequate antibiotics use is indispensable.

With this in mind, the aims of this chapter are:

- To review the major antibiotic classes discovered and their mechanisms of action;

- To discuss the relevance of an adequate antibiotic use and highlight the main barriers associated with the emergence of ABR;

- To describe the importance of establishing good pharmacovigilance practices;

- To summarize available epidemiological data concerning antibiotic use related ADR;

- To analyze the reports received by the EudraVigilance system regarding the exclusive usage of antibiotics.

2. Antibiotics

The global significance of antibiotics discovery in medical science is unquestionable. According to the Centers for Disease Control and Prevention (CDC), antibiotics can be described as "medicines that fight infections caused by bacteria in humans and animals, by either killing the bacteria or making it difficult for the bacteria to grow and multiply" [13]. Antibiotics can be of natural occurring origin or chemically synthesized, and have proven to be essential in fighting infectious diseases [14]. The discovery and development of these compounds has allowed the effective treatment of several bacterial infections, leading to an increased lifespan and to an improvement in the quality of life of millions of people [14].

Salvarsan, the first synthetic anti-infective drug reported, was synthesized and discovered by Paul Ehrlich, Alfred Bertheim and Sahachiro Hata in 1907. This antibiotic had its first clinical application in 1910 in syphilis treatment, and was shown to be highly effective and therapeutically safe, regardless of the side effects [1, 15, 16]. Afterwards, in 1932, Gerhard Domagk discovered Prontosil, a sulfonamide drug, which was further developed and commercially released in 1935 for public use by the pharmaceutical company Bayer. These were two of the first antibiotics of synthetic origin discovered [14–16]. On the other hand, penicillin was the first naturally occurring antibiotic discovered in modern medicine, being observed in a petri dish in 1928 by Alexander Fleming. In 1941, Howard Florey, Norman Heatly and Ernst Chain pursued Fleming's studies and penicillin was finally produced in sufficient quantities to be used in clinical trials, allowing the treatment of uncountable soldiers during World War II. In 1945, the discovery of this unprecedent live-saving antibiotic led Fleming, Florey and Chain to won the Nobel prize [1, 14–16].

The discovery of these three antibacterial drug agents was remarkable and unveiled the future discovery, development and release of several new antibiotic classes during the so called "Golden Age" of antibiotics, a period between 1940s and middle 1960s [1, 15]. Interestingly, most of the antibiotics discovered during this era are still being currently used in the treatment of bacterial infections, once the pharmaceutical industry significantly reduced its investments in the production of new antibiotics due to the little benefit over existing treatments [3].

Antibiotics are classified in different classes. Some share similar chemical and pharmacological features and thus are used in the treatment of similar bacteria infections. These classes briefly comprise β-lactams, sulfonamides, aminoglycosides, tetracyclines, chloramphenicol, macrolides, glycopeptides, sulphonamides, ansamycins, polymyxins, quinolones, streptogramins, oxazolidinones and lipopeptides [16].

According to the Anatomical Therapeutic Chemical (ATC) Index 2020 from the WHO Collaborating Centre for Drug Statistics Methodology Norwegian Institute of Public Health, antibiotics are categorized as antibacterials for systemic use – J01 therapeutic subgroup, belong to the anti-infectives for systemic use (J anatomical group) and consist of the 10 different pharmacological subgroups displayed in **Table 1** [17]. Additionally, antibiotics can also be categorized as bactericidal or bacteriostatic, based on their mechanism of action (**Table 1**). The general assumption within the society for many years was that bactericidal antibiotics (agents that eliminate bacteria by causing cell death) were more powerful and effective than bacteriostatic antibiotics (agents that inhibit bacterial growth and reproduction). However, it became relevant to assess if this belief was indeed true and verified at a clinical level for several bacterial infections [18]. Several studies included in a systematic literature review on the topic have shown that for many invasive bacterial infections, such as pneumonia, skin and soft tissue infection, intraabdominal, genital and nonendocarditis bloodstream infections, there was no significant clinical differences in outcomes nor in mortality. Therefore, one can assume that this classification seems to be irrelevant when applied to these types of clinical infections [18].

2.1 Main challenges with antibiotic use

The discovery of new antibiotics allowed to save countless lives and revolutionize the future of medicine concerning, for instance, transplantation, surgery and chemotherapy, by preventing and treating bacterial infections in these patients. This has led to a significant decline in mortality and morbidity, and to an extended expected lifespan worldwide [19].

After this remarkable era, only a couple of new antibiotic classes were discovered, and the ones that were in clinical use started to become less effective, due to the rise of an emerging and global health threat, the ABR [7, 19].

The development of ABR is created by specific modifications in bacteria, namely mutations or acquisition of resistant genes by horizontal gene-transfer, allowing them to proliferate and survive in the presence of an antibiotic concentration that used to be enough to either prevent the growth or completely eliminate these

J01: Antibacterials for systemic use				
ATC code	**Pharmacological subgroup**	**Examples of antibiotics**	**Type of agent**	**Mechanism of action**
J01A	Tetracyclines	• Demeclocycline • Doxycycline • Chlortetracycline • Lymecycline • Metacycline • Oxytetracycline • Tetracycline • Minocycline	Bacteriostatic	Bacterial protein biosynthesis inhibition (30-S ribosomal subunit targeting)
J01B	Amphenicols	• Chloramphenicol • Thiamphenicol • Combinations of Thiamphenicol	Bacteriostatic	Bacterial protein biosynthesis inhibition (50-S ribosomal subunit targeting)
J01C	β-Lactam Antibacterials – Penicillins	• Ampicillin • Amoxicillin • Benzylpenicillin • Flucloxacillin • Meticillin • Sulbactam • Combinations of penicillins	Bactericidal	Bacterial cell wall synthesis inhibition
J01D	Other β-Lactam Antibacterials	• Cephalosporins: Cefalexin, Cefoxitin, Cefotaxime, Cefepime • Monobactams: Aztreonam • Carbapenems: Meropenem • Other cephalosporins and penems: Ceftobiprole medocaril	Bactericidal	Bacterial cell wall synthesis inhibition
J01E	Sulfonamides and Trimethoprim	• Trimethoprim • Sulfanilamide • Sulfadiazine • Sulfadimethoxine • Combinations of Sulfonamides and Trimethoprim	Bacteriostatic	Folic acid synthesis inhibition
J01F	Macrolides, Lincosamides and Streptogramins	• Macrolides: Erythromycin, Azythromycin • Lincosamides: Clindamycin, Lincomycin • Streptogramins: Pristinamycin, Quinupristin/Dalfopristin	Bacteriostatic (Macrolides and Lincosamides) and Bactericidal (Streptogramins)	Bacterial protein biosynthesis inhibition (50-S ribosomal subunit targeting)

J01: Antibacterials for systemic use				
ATC code	**Pharmacological subgroup**	**Examples of antibiotics**	**Type of agent**	**Mechanism of action**
J01G	Aminoglycoside Antibacterials	• Streptomycins: Streptomycin, Streptoduocin • Other Aminoglycosides: Neomycin, Kanamycin, Gentamicin	Bactericidal	Bacterial protein biosynthesis inhibition (30-S ribosomal subunit targeting)
J01M	Quinolone Antibacterials	• Fluoroquinolones: Ciprofloxacin, Levofloxacin, Trovafloxacin • Other Quinolones: Nalidixic acid, Cinoxacin, Oxolinic acid	Bactericidal	Nucleic acid synthesis inhibition (inhibitors of DNA replication)
J01R	Combinations of Antibacterials	• Penicillins with other Antibacterials • Sulfonamides with other Antibacterials • Spiramycin and Metronidazole • Tetracycline and Oleandomycin • Ciprofloxacin and Ornidazole • Norfloxacin and Tinidazole	Bacteriostatic and Bactericidal	Multiple mechanisms inhibition
J01X	Other Antibacterials	• Glycopeptide Antibacterials: Vancomycin • Polymyxins: Colistin • Steroid Antibacterials: Fusidic acid • Imidazole Derivatives: Metronidazole • Nitrofuran Derivatives: Nitrofurantoin • Other Antibacterials: Fosfomycin	Bacteriostatic and Bactericidal	Multiple mechanisms inhibition

Table 1.
Classification of antibiotics based on the ATC index 2020.

microorganisms [4]. The ABR phenomenon brought serious health and financial consequences to the society, particularly the increased risk in compromising the healthcare sector, together with a global economic impact, because the pharmaceutical companies no longer perceived both antibiotic discovery and development as lucrative investments [19]. Over the past 25 years, several economic, regulatory, and scientific barriers arose and led to a significant decline in the production of new antibiotics, with only two new classes entering the market and being applied into clinical therapy. Instead of generating new drug classes chemically different from the existent ones, the pharmaceutical industry chose to modify the already existent antibiotics, particularly the naturally-occurring antibiotics, and to alert for its judicious use, aiming to increase their treatment efficiency and combat bacterial resistance on the long run [14, 20].

The global prevalence of bacteria resistance to antibiotics has been progressively growing. The major facilitating drivers of ABR are the overuse and misuse of these drugs, both in human and veterinary medicine and agriculture, as well as the inappropriate prescription of antibiotic therapy by health professionals. Additionally, ABR can also be triggered by the excessive and unrestricted consumption of antibiotics easily available at low price and over the counter for self-medication, in countries that lack antibiotic regulations, or by the free online acquisition of these medicines in countries where antibiotics are strictly regulated [4, 5, 19].

When an antibiotic successfully reaches its target with a certain required concentration, it causes the death or growth inhibition of pathogens. The resistance mechanisms frequently used by bacteria can be developed by the modification of the antibiotic main target or by the reduction of the antibiotic quantity able to reach the target. There are four key molecular mechanisms involved in bacteria resistance [21]:

- Antibiotic modification or destruction – production of specific enzymes able to inhibit or destroy the drug through chemical alterations, thus preventing the antibiotic to interact with its target;

- Antibiotic uptake decrease and/or antibiotic extruding via efflux pumps – leads to a significant reduction in antibiotic's intracellular concentration, preventing it from achieving the target site;

- Target sites modification – either by protecting (antibiotic is unable to achieve its binding site) and/or modifying (the affinity between the drug and its target is reduced) the target site;

- Bacterial resistance development due to global cell adaptive procedures – bacteria are able to survive and protect the disruption of essential cellular mechanisms, by developing resistance inside the host environment.

2.2 Epidemiological data

A close link between excessive and inadequate antibiotic consumption and the associated ABR spread has been extensively reported in the literature as a public health hazard worldwide. Antibiotics overuse and misuse were shown to be two of the most critical ABR contributors [5, 19, 20].

The 2019 annual epidemiological report of antimicrobial consumption in the EU/European Economic Area (EEA) published by the ECDC disclosed that the average total consumption of antibacterials for systemic use (ATC group J01) from both primary care and hospital sectors in 2018 was of 19.4 defined daily doses (DDD) per 1000 inhabitants per day (ranging from 9.5 in the Netherlands to 34.1 in Greece). This surveillance report is based on antimicrobial consumption data reported by the 28 EU Member States, together with 2 EEA countries (namely, Iceland and Norway). Overall, a statistically significant decrease in the trend of antibiotics consumption over the 10-year period (2009–2019) was observed in the EU/EEA, with statistically significant differences (either a decrease or an increase) being noticed for particular countries. Apart from Slovakia, the antibiotic subgroup with the highest average consumption in all countries of the EU/EEA was β-lactam antibacterials – Penicillins (J01C) [22].

Approximately two-thirds of the world's population are living at the Asia Pacific region (APAC), one of the largest vulnerable regions to the serious problems posed by ABR. Countries belonging to the WHO South-East Asia region were acknowledged to display the greatest risk of ABR development and propagation comparing to all WHO regions [23]. The lack of a formal and efficient surveillance system, strictly dedicated to detecting and monitor human antibiotic consumption and resistance in APAC countries, makes it impossible to determine the overall burden and estimates of antibiotic use in this region. Nevertheless, there is a high demand for the adoption of successful strategies aiming to decrease the impact of this public health threat in Asia, as it is one of the most critical ABR epicenters worldwide [23].

Data on total antibiotic consumption in DDD per 1000 inhabitants per day are presented for 2 Asian and 1 African countries of the WHO Eastern Mediterranean Region, respectively the Islamic Republic of Iran with 38.8 (wholesalers data), and Jordan with 8.9 (import data, with the exception of locally produced medicines that would account for a significant fraction of the total antibiotic use), as well as Sudan with 35.3 (combined data from import and local manufacturers). The antibiotic subgroup most commonly used in Islamic Republic of Iran and Sudan was penicillin, respectively accounting for 33% and 41% of the total consumption, while in Jordan more than 50% of the antibiotics consumed were macrolides/lincosamides/streptogramins (J01F), followed by penicillins and other β-lactam antibacterials (J01D) [24].

The same data is also available for 6 countries of the WHO Western Pacific Region, including Brunei Darussalam with 5.9 DDD per 1000 inhabitants per day, Japan with 14.2, Mongolia with 64.4, New Zealand with 22.7, Philippines with 8.2 and the Republic of Korea with 27.7. However, Brunei Darussalam and New Zealand only provided partial data, either of the public health care or community sectors, respectively [24]. Overall, within this region, approximately 33 to 50% of the antibiotics used were penicillins. The most commonly consumed antibiotic subgroups in Brunei Darussalam, Japan, Mongolia, New Zealand, Philippines and Republic of Korea were, respectively, β-lactam antibacterials (70%), macrolides/lincosamides/streptogramins (32%) and other β-lactam antibacterials (32%), penicillins (33%), penicillins (44%), tetracyclines (J01A, 30%) and penicillins (30%) and other β-lactam antibacterials (33%) [24].

The WHO African Region only provided total antibiotic consumption data in DDD per 1000 inhabitants per day for 4 countries, specifically Burkina Faso with 13.8, Burundi with 4.4 (data restricted to the public sector), Côte d'Ivoire with 10.7 and, finally, the United Republic of Tanzania with 27.3 (data reports only from 2016). The pharmacological subgroup most commonly consumed in all these 4 countries was penicillin, accounting for about 40% of the total consumption in both Burkina Faso and Côte d'Ivoire, 78% in Burundi and 27% in United Republic of Tanzania [24].

The ABR threat greatly affects healthcare development, food production, and lifespan. To efficiently combat ABR, the 1st step is to prevent bacterial infections, the 2nd step is to restrict the resistant bacteria spread by improving an adequate antibiotic use and, finally, the 3rd step is to immediately interrupt the spread when the development has occurred [25].

According to the CDC's Antibiotic Resistance Threats in the United States (US) Report from 2019, which delivered the most recent national antibiotic resistance-associated burden estimates, there are still over 2.8 million infections occurring in the US per year, yielding more than 350 thousand deaths. Although estimates have improved, particularly the death rate which decreased by 18% when compared to the same report from 2013, the high number of ABR-associated infections still remains an important challenge [25]. Moreover, 2016 CDC estimates revealed that approximately 30% of all antibiotics prescribed in the US, which corresponds to about 47 million prescriptions per year, are still being inadequately used to treat diseases that do not require antibiotics [26].

Since ABR is a natural and irreversible phenomenon, it is crucial that countries around the world start adopting rigorous measures to slow down and inhibit the spread of bacterial resistance. In response to the emerging global public health threat posed by ABR, a number of national and international actions and initiatives have been developed in recent years to address this issue [27]. In 2015, WHO adopted a global action plan with several interventions that included strengthening health systems and surveillance, reducing the unnecessary use of antibiotics, as well as the prevention and control of ABR in humans, animals, agriculture, and the environment, highlighting the need for an efficient, indispensable and global "OneHealth" approach [27–29]. According to the CDC, the "OneHealth" approach is a "collaborative, multisectoral, and transdisciplinary approach—working at the local, regional, national, and global levels—with the goal of achieving optimal health outcomes recognizing the interconnection between people, animals, plants, and their shared environment" [30]. Subsequently, on June 29th, 2017, the European Commission adopted a similar integrated action plan, consisting of a series of global, rigorous and high priority strategies and measures, designed to restrict the development and spread of ABR in humans and animals, based on the "OneHealth" perspective [31]. Antibiotic resistance is indeed a One Health challenge, where people's and animal's health are linked together with the environment, that must be rapidly curbed.

The pointless or inadequate antibiotics usage is frequently determined by the knowledge, attitudes and beliefs of all the involved stakeholders on this relevant topic. In order to fight this threat, a couple of initiatives have been adopted by many countries worldwide. These have shown to effectively impact ABR and comprise bacterial infection regulatory programs to limit the transmission of resistant microorganisms, antibiotic stewardship courses based on the adherence to awareness guidelines and approaches to increase the judicious antibiotic prescription, educational interventions among health professionals to improve prudent antibiotic prescription and vaccination programs [20, 29, 32–35].

3. Adverse drug reactions associated with antibiotics

Pharmacovigilance is very important for monitoring the safety profile of authorized drugs [12, 36]. The ADR remain a challenge in medicine use and are regarded as a critical public health concern due to their potential harmful life-threatening effects [37].

According to the European Directive 2010/84/EU, an *adverse reaction* is defined as a "response to a medicinal product which is noxious and unintended". Moreover, these reactions may arise from the use of the medicinal product within or outside the terms of the marketing authorization (such as off-label use, overdose, misuse, abuse) or from occupational exposure. On the other hand, the definition of an *adverse effect* is given by the EU Directive 2001/20/EC as "any untoward medical occurrence in a patient or clinical trial subject administered a medicinal product and which does not necessarily have a causal relationship with this treatment". One can then conclude that while an adverse effect is not necessarily triggered by the drug, as it is only temporally correlated with the drug use, an ADR is a form of adverse effect both temporally and causally associated with the drug [38, 39].

The classical or traditional pharmacological classification of ADR primarily adopted was only differentiating dose-related and non-dose-related reactions, respectively as type A and type B, being solely characterized by properties of the drug (its well-known pharmacology and dose dependent effects). Subsequently, other 4 types of reactions were further established to facilitate the inclusion of adverse reactions that did not belong to type A or type B. Therefore, the modern ADR classification currently includes 6 types of reactions [40].

In 2003, to improve the drawbacks and oversimplifications of the traditional approach, an alternative and more accurate classification system was proposed by Aronson and Ferner, as it had been noticed that some ADR still did not fit well into just one of the classes described above. This classification scheme is known as DoTS and operates by taking into account 3 major parameters: the Dose responsiveness of the drug, the Time course of the reaction and the relevant Susceptibility factors of the patient (including genetic, pathological and other biological differences). Although this 3-dimensional approach is more precise and comprehensive when considering the diagnosis and prevention of ADR, it is also more complex for daily use, which prevented its extensive use in the clinic [41].

Globally, ADR have shown to cause significant morbidity and mortality across diverse populations, either in hospitalized or ambulatory patients, with a significant economic burden to the healthcare system. Adverse reactions affect the quality of life of patients, their confidence in the healthcare system and can significantly increase hospitalizations and the hospital stay period [42, 43].

Over the years, several studies have reported that on average, ADR are responsible for 5–10% of the hospitalizations worldwide, with 80% being frequently considered predictable and possibly avoidable reactions (type A). Moreover, it has also been shown that approximately one fourth of the ambulatory patients in primary care centers can also suffer an ADR reported as serious in 13% of the cases [42].

Studies from the US have shown that ADR were observed in over 1.2 million hospital stays (about 3.1% of all hospital stays) in 2004. In US hospitals, the incidence of serious and fatal ADR was extremely high, with evaluations of 6.7% and 0.32% respectively, making ADR between the 4th and 6th leading cause of death. In 2012, a management consulting firm estimated a profit of USD 115 billion for the prevention of 35 million adverse drug events. In United Kingdom, ADR incidence among admitted patients was found to be 6.5%, with admissions costing up to £466 million annually or 0.62% of annual health budget [44]. Within the EU, in 2008 the European Commission estimated that around 5% of all hospital admissions were triggered by ADR, with 5% of hospitalized patients experiencing an ADR during their hospital stay. Additionally, approximately 197 thousand deaths per year took place in the EU due to ADR [43].

These findings were undoubtedly one of the starting points for the implementation of a new EU pharmacovigilance regulatory framework in 2012, to reduce the ADR burden [43]. Currently, countless countries around the world already have well-established, active and robust national pharmacovigilance systems to safeguard patient's wellbeing.

Some medicines have been especially involved in hospital admissions due to ADR, including antibiotics. Inpatients are given at least one antibiotic in about 50% of the cases, with roughly 20–30% of these being considered unnecessary and accounting for 20–50% of drug costs in hospitals [10, 45]. Additionally, a previous study has reported that although antibiotics use seems to lead to a small incidence of adverse events, its widespread consumption accounts for 23% of all adverse events documented [10]. Between 2000 and 2010, developing countries were the major contributors to the global rise in antibiotics use and, consequently, in the risk of acquiring associated ADR [11].

There is a lack of studies assessing the incidence of ADR due to antibiotic consumption in the hospital sector, during patient's admission, stay and after discharge, as well as its incidence across all antibiotic classes. Nevertheless, the available literature has shown the clear contribution of antibiotics to 19% of ADR in the emergency department in the US between 2004 and 2006 (with allergic reactions accounting for 79%), 8% linked to hospital admissions in Greece in 2005, 6% in Spain between 2001 and 2006, 5% in The Netherlands in 2003, and 11% in India between 2002 and 2009, together with 10% of hospital-acquired ADR in the US and 22% in South Africa [11].

There are several mechanisms explaining different ADR, and the most well-known include pharmacological causes, idiosyncrasies, hypersensitivity (allergic reactions), carcinogenesis and teratogenesis, direct toxicity, chronic exposure, drug-disease interaction and drug intolerance [46].

3.1 ADR analysis in Europe: EudraVigilance

EudraVigilance, the official EU pharmacovigilance database managing the collection and analysis of suspected ADR to authorized medical products in the EEA, was primarily launched in 2001, with a new format emerging in 2017. This new revised and enhanced version aimed to achieve an improved effective monitoring of the medicine safety, contributing to public health protection, and the communication of validated signals to the European Medicines Agency (EMA) and the national medicines regulatory authorities, in line with the legislative framework. By the end of 2017, submissions to EudraVigilance overcome the 12 million individual case safety reports (ICSR), referring to around 8 million individual cases, and making it one of the largest spontaneous reporting systems worldwide [47].

As previously mentioned, one of the drug classes most commonly prescribed and responsible for ADR, both in primary care and hospital sectors, are antibiotics. For Portugal, according to the data provided by the System of Information and Monitoring of the Portuguese National Health System (SIM@SNS) platform [48], developed by the shared services of the Health Ministry, the four antibacterials for systemic use mostly prescribed during the last couple of years (2018–2020) were: a combination of Amoxicillin and Clavulanic acid (**I**), Azithromycin (**II**), Amoxicillin (**III**) and Fosfomycin (**IV**) [49]. In particular, during the year of 2019, the total number of antibiotic packages prescribed within the public sector accounted for around 4.5 million, from which 1.27, 0.63, 0.52, and 0.35 million, respectively corresponded to I, II, III and IV. Data from 2018 revealed the same trend as 2019. Until August 2020, the only alteration observed was the increase in fosfomycin prescriptions over amoxicillin [49].

The individual safety reports stored at the VigiBase (for I) [50] and EudraVigilance (for II, III and IV) [51] databases at 14th November 2020 revealed that among all ADR reported, the most affected System Organ Classes (SOC) for each antibiotic were[1]:

I. Combination of Amoxicillin and Clavulanic Acid (ICSR total = 140942): Skin and subcutaneous tissue disorders – **50.5%**, Gastrointestinal disorders – **24.9%**, and General disorders and administration site conditions – **11.9%**. Within all ADR reported for this combination, 24.6% were considered serious ADR;

[1] The antibiotic-associated ADR reported data are displayed in different ways, as they were retrieved from two different databases, VigiBase (for I) and EudraVigilance (for II, III and IV).

II. Azithromycin (ICSR total = 13404): Gastrointestinal disorders – **26.2%** (of which 15.6% were serious), Skin and subcutaneous tissue disorders – **24.7%** (of which 17% were serious) and General disorders and administration site conditions – **24.5%** (of which 20.2% were serious);

III. Amoxicillin (ICSR total = 34427): Skin and subcutaneous tissue disorders – **56.2%** (of which 36% were serious), Gastrointestinal disorders – **18.4%** (of which 10.9% were serious) and General disorders and administration site conditions – **16.1%** (of which 11.8% were serious);

IV. Fosfomycin (ICSR total = 2483): Gastrointestinal disorders – **38.6%** (of which 10.1% were serious), Skin and subcutaneous tissue disorders – **24.8%** (of which 12.6% were serious) and General disorders and administration site conditions – **21.3%** (of which 11.2% were serious).

The most common ADR reported within each SOC caused by the consumption of these antibiotics include rash, urticaria and pruritus for skin and subcutaneous tissue disorders, diarrhea, nausea, vomiting and abdominal pain for gastrointestinal disorder and pyrexia, malaise, fatigue and asthenia for general disorders and administration condition sites.

The use of antibiotics can result in ADR, among which hypersensitivity reactions. One of the safest and more effective antibiotic subgroups is the β-lactam antibacterials. Within this subgroup, penicillin is one of the most prescribed antibiotics worldwide and is frequently associated with reported allergic reactions. Around 10% of the global population report an allergy to β-lactams, leading to an increased use of broad-spectrum antibiotics, promoting the risk for the development of resistant bacteria and adverse effects, together with an increased cost. Most reports of penicillin allergy describe an unknown or a mild cutaneous reaction. The estimated frequency of the more serious anaphylactic reactions to penicillin is roughly 0.02% to 0.04%, being rarer after oral or cutaneous exposure [52].

3.2 Special populations: children, pregnant women and older adults

ADR reporting system databases are of great utility in the early detection of medicine safety issues [8]. Most of the available data regarding ADR prevalence refer to adult populations within a hospital context [53]. Thereby, it is extremely important to increase our knowledge and perception on ADR incidence in special populations, such as the pediatric (0–18 years old), pregnant women and older adults (≥ 65 years old), as they may differ regarding the most frequently involved drugs and ADR manifestations, and may be at an increased risk due to their general exclusion from pre-marketing clinical assays.

3.2.1 Children

Antibiotics are among the most commonly prescribed drugs in children. Reports from a study conducted in the US during 2016 revealed that 47.4% of infants between 0 and 4 years old received at least one antibiotic prescription, when compared to 39.8% of the adult population. Although these drugs are very valuable for the treatment of severe infection diseases, its high and inadequate consumption can frequently lead to an increased bacterial resistance, as well as to the occurrence of adverse effects even if mild and spontaneously resolving [54]. Antibiotics have been repeatedly reported as the leading contributors to ADR in children. Children can be at an increased risk due to their anatomical and physiological characteristics, such as their immature immune systems, especially in the first years of life. Moreover, there is a frequent abuse and misuse of these drugs in pediatric clinical practice due to lack of pharmacokinetics data or dose-finding studies, and many antibiotics are prescribed on an unlicensed or "off-label" basis as they were only tested and authorized for adults. Although many adverse events are equal in children and adults, with age not contributing to the frequency and severity of the ADR, there are a few number of antibiotic-associated ADR depending on the unique pharmacokinetic and pharmacodynamic features of the antibiotic that can differ significantly with age, particularly when administered to newborns and infants [54].

A systematic review [55] of ADR in pediatric patients reported that the overall rates of hospital admissions caused by ADR ranged from 0.4% to 10.3% of all children, while the ADR incidence rate varied between 0.6% and 16.8% among children exposed to a drug during hospital stay [8, 53]. Furthermore, a study performed between 2011 and 2015 in the US, based on 6542 surveillance cases, estimated that approximately 70 thousand annual emergency department visits were made for antibiotic-associated ADR among children. This review also showed that the antibiotic most commonly associated with ADR was, by far, the oral penicillin (55.7%), and the most typical clinical manifestations attributed to antibiotics were allergic reactions. Within the pediatric population, amoxicillin was found to be the antibiotic most frequently implicated among children under 10 years old [56]. The findings obtained from ADR reports of two studies conducted within the Portuguese pediatric population between 2003 and 2012 (age range 0–17 years old) and 2006 and 2016 (age range 10–18 years old) demonstrated that the most representative ADR identified involved the subsequent top 4 SOC: general disorders and administration site conditions, followed by skin and subcutaneous tissue reactions, nervous system disorders and gastrointestinal disorders. Antibacterials for systemic use were the second most represented group after vaccines [8, 53].

The individual safety reports stored at the VigiBase (for I) [50] and EudraVigilance (for II, III and IV) [51] databases revealed that, among all ADR reported specifically for children, the percentage of antibiotic-associated ADR for the antibiotics mostly prescribed in Portugal between 2018 and 2020 was of **16.6%** for **I** (combination of amoxicillin and clavulanic acid), **17.1%** for **II** (azithromycin), **17.7%** for **III** (amoxicillin) and **4.2%** for **IV** (fosfomycin). Moreover, the most affected SOC were[2]:

II. ICSR total = 2297: Skin and subcutaneous tissue disorders – **35%**, Gastrointestinal disorders – **25%** and General disorders and administration site conditions – **19.5%**;

III. ICSR total = 6105: Skin and subcutaneous tissue disorders – **69.3%**, Gastrointestinal disorders – **16.9%** and General disorders and administration site conditions – **14.1%**;

IV. ICSR total = 107: Gastrointestinal disorders – **27.1%**, Skin and subcutaneous tissue disorders – **25.2%** and General disorders and administration site conditions – **22.4%**.

3.2.2 Pregnant women

People are aware about the existent lack of information concerning drug safety during pregnancy, mainly because pregnant women are often excluded from trials

[2] SOC data for the combination of amoxicillin and clavulanic acid (I) were not available at VigiBase.

throughout the clinical development of the drug. Since 1980, estimates indicate that only 10% of the authorized drugs have enough data involving child risk in pregnancy. Thus, there is a high need for epidemiological studies in pregnant women aiming to evaluate the incidence of ADR [57].

Since there are no reports of totally innocuous drugs commercially available, pregnant women must be cautious and try to avoid, as much as possible, the consumption of medicines, particularly during the first trimester, and only use them when the benefits to the mother outweigh the fetus risk [58]. Over the last years, it has been observed a rise in the number of women consuming drugs during pregnancy. Antibiotics are among one of the classes most commonly prescribed to treat infections in pregnant women, constituting nearly 80% of all drugs prescription, of which roughly 1 in every 4 women consume at least one antibiotic throughout their pregnancy course. However, its use must be prudent as the first concern is to protect the fetus from potential ADR resulting from antibiotic use [57, 58]. Urinary tract infections, sexually transmitted infections and upper respiratory tract infections represent 3 of the most typical infectious diseases found during pregnancy. When not treated, urinary tract and sexually transmitted infections represent an important risk to the fetus with consequences such as, as low birth weight, prematurity and spontaneous abortion. Moreover, the risk for short-term (congenital abnormalities) and long-term (changes in the gut microbiome, asthma, atopic disease) effects in the newborn, and physiological changes that usually take place during pregnancy, have also been related to antibiotic therapy [57].

Overall, there are several antibiotics that can be generally used during pregnancy without compromising safety, such as β-lactams (with penicillin and derivatives being the most prescribed drugs to pregnant women), vancomycin, macrolides, clindamycin, and fosfomycin, and others that must be mostly avoided, such as fluoroquinolones and tetracyclines [57]. In fact, penicillins have a long safety track record during pregnancy, but are usually substituted by macrolides as alternative for patients with penicillin allergies. Very recently, a cohort population-based study from UK has shown that the prescription of macrolides instead of penicillin antibiotics led to an enhanced risk of major malformation, primarily those derived from the cardiovascular system, but only over the first pregnancy trimester. This study also reported an enhanced risk of genital malformations linked to macrolides prescription in any trimester, advertising for the careful use of this antibiotic subgroup in pregnant women [59]. Some studies have also indicated an increased asthma risk in early childhood, as well as an increased risk of childhood epilepsy and obesity linked to antibiotic use during pregnancy [58].

The use of 3 of the most prescribed antibiotics in Portugal over the last years, namely amoxicillin clavulanate, amoxicillin and fosfomycin, has been considered safe and well-tolerated during pregnancy, with no adverse effects being shown in the fetus or infant [57].

3.2.3 Older adults

Infectious diseases in the elderly population remains a public health concern because of the high mortality and morbidity outcomes. The geriatric population, regarded as a special population by the International Council for Harmonization (ICH), is more prone to develop ADR because they usually exhibit a combination of increased critical risk factors that can promote these reactions. These risk factors comprise multimorbidity, polypharmacy, changes in medication adherence, pharmacokinetics, greater vulnerability, aging-related physiological changes (changes in the body mass distribution, renal function, metabolic capacity and alteration in blood protein levels), deficit in the immune system, weakening cognition, in addition to a clear lack on drug use information in the older people [60]. Research studies have estimated an ADR risk in older adults of four times higher than the rest of the population. Old age is also a critical factor for extended hospital stays, enhanced prevalence of complication and falls. The large majority of reported ADR in the older adults belong to type A, possibly avoidable and linked to commonly prescribed drugs. Common geriatric syndromes from older adults include delirium, falls, dizziness, urinary incontinence, which can sometimes be mistaken with typical manifestations from older people. Therefore, given their heterogeneity, to efficiently prevent the high ADR incidence in the older people, it is essential to focus on person-centered care intervention allied to good clinical practice [60].

Between 2007 and 2009, data from an US report on hospitalizations after emergency department visits for adverse events revealed that 3.8% of the total hospitalizations were due to the use of antimicrobial agents. In fact, these agents were the 5th most common treatment class involved in hospitalizations. Data showed that the most frequent clinical adverse event manifestations arisen from antimicrobials use leading to hospitalizations were allergic reactions (36.2%), dyspnea and weakness (22.5%), gastrointestinal effects (20.5%), and neurologic effects (18.3%). Some of these adverse events, such as dyspnea, weakness, neurological adverse events, and effects on blood pressure may potentially promote significant negative implications in older patients, leading to altered mental status, falls, and hypotension [61].

The individual safety reports stored at the VigiBase (for I) [50] and EudraVigilance (for II, III and IV) [51] databases revealed that, among all ADR reported specifically for older adults (≥ 65 years old), the percentage of antibiotic-associated ADR for the antibiotics mostly prescribed in Portugal between 2018 and 2020 was of **22.7%** for **I** (combination of amoxicillin and clavulanic acid), **20.7%** for **II** (azithromycin), **22.7%** for **III** (amoxicillin) and **31.5%** for **IV** (fosfomycin). Moreover, the most affected SOC were[3]:

II. ICSR total = 2767: General disorders and administration site conditions – **26.5%**, Gastrointestinal disorders – **21.5%** and Skin and subcutaneous tissue disorders – **21%**;

III. ICSR total = 7813: Skin and subcutaneous tissue disorders – **47.8%**, Gastrointestinal disorders – **18%** and General disorders and administration site conditions – **16.5%**;

IV. ICSR total = 780: Gastrointestinal disorders – **33.2%**, Skin and subcutaneous tissue disorders – **27.1%** and General disorders and administration site conditions – **21.8%**.

4. Conclusions

Overall, antibiotics are undoubtedly among the most successful drug agents in the world. They are attributed to having improved patient care and revolutionized modern medicine. However, the inappropariate prescribing of these agents has led to the development of one of the biggest public health concern: antimicrobial resistances [4, 5]. Therefore, it is vital to understand and overcome the main barriers and challenges resulting from antibiotics usage, aiming to design and develop educational interventions for increase awareness and knowledge within the society, and hopefully be able to change people's and prescribing physician's behavior.

[3] SOC data for the combination of amoxicillin and clavulanic acid (**I**) were not available at VigiBase.

Pharmacovigilance is a global top priority in healthcare systems. It provides instruments for monitoring the safety of medicines on the market through prevention, detection and assessment of adverse reactions, as well as invaluable information on the benefit/risk ratio of a health product throughout its life cycle [12, 36].

Currently, ADR are still ranked among the leading mortality causes in many countries and are recognize as hazards of drug therapy [42, 43]. Although ADR are prevalent in all ages, it is more difficult to predict the effect of the drugs among the special populations that do not take part in clinical trials. Post-marketing surveillance through pharmacovigilance centers is extremely important and the most efficient way to monitor ADR, especially for those groups [12, 42].

Although antibiotics are considered safe when rationally used for treatment and prophylaxis of several infectious diseases, with its prescription being generally high among all ages, these drugs can also substantially contribute to reported ADR, especially β-lactam antibacterials, and macrolides [10, 11, 45]. The most affected organ systems involved are the gastrointestinal system and the skin.

In sum, a visible reduction in global human mortality and morbidity, as well as in health costs, would certainly be noticed with the implementation of international and national campaigns alerting to both the rational use of antibiotics and the importance of reporting ADR, aiming to minimize patient's harm and significantly improve public health.

Acknowledgements

This research was funded by the project, PTDC/SAU-SER/31678/2017, supported by the operational program on competitiveness and internationalization (POCI) in its FEDER/FNR component, POCI-01-0145-FEDER-031678, and by the Foundation for Science and Technology in its state budget component (OE).

Conflict of interest

The authors declare no conflict of interest.

Appendices and nomenclature

ABR	Antibiotic Resistance
ADR	Adverse Drug Reactions
APAC	Asia Pacific region
ATC	Anatomical Therapeutic Chemical
CDC	Centers for Disease Control and Prevention
DDD	Defined Daily Doses
EARS-Net	European Antimicrobial Resistance Surveillance Network
EEA	European Economic Area
EMA	European Medicines Agency
EU	European Union
ICH	International Council for Harmonization
ICSR	Individual Case Safety Report
SOC	System Organ Classes
US	United States
WHO	World Health Organization

Author details

Tânia Magalhães Silva[1], Eva Rebelo Gomes[2], Inês Ribeiro-Vaz[3,4], Fátima Roque[5,6] and Maria Teresa Herdeiro[1*]

1 iBiMED - Institute of Biomedicine, Department of Medical Sciences, University of Aveiro, Aveiro, Portugal

2 Allergy and Clinical Immunology Service, University Hospital Center of Porto, Porto, Portugal

3 Porto Pharmacovigilance Centre, Faculty of Medicine of University of Porto, Porto, Portugal

4 Center for Health Technology and Services Research (CINTESIS), Faculty of Medicine of University of Porto, Porto, Portugal

5 Research Unit for Inland Development, Guarda Polytechnic Institute (UDI-IPG), Guarda, Portugal

6 Health Sciences Research Centre, University of Beira Interior (CICS-UBI), Covilhã, Portugal

*Address all correspondence to: teresaherdeiro@ua.pt

References

[1] Hutchings MI, Truman AW, Wilkinson B. Antibiotics: past, present and future. *Curr Opin Microbiol* 2019; 51: 72-80.

[2] World Health Organization. Antibiotic Resistance, https://www.who.int/news-room/fact-sheets/detail/antibiotic-resistance (2020, accessed 26 October 2020).

[3] Fernandes P, Martens E. Antibiotics in late clinical development. *Biochem Pharmacol* 2017; 133: 152-163.

[4] Sabtu N, Enoch DA, Brown NM. Antibiotic resistance: what, why, where, when and how? *Br Med Bull* 2015; ldv041.

[5] Machowska A, Stålsby Lundborg C. Drivers of Irrational Use of Antibiotics in Europe. *Int J Environ Res Public Health* 2018; 16: 27.

[6] Cassini A, Högberg LD, Plachouras D, et al. Attributable deaths and disability-adjusted life-years caused by infections with antibiotic-resistant bacteria in the EU and the European Economic Area in 2015: a population-level modelling analysis. *Lancet Infect Dis* 2019; 19: 56-66.

[7] Prestinaci F, Pezzotti P, Pantosti A. Antimicrobial resistance: a global multifaceted phenomenon. *Pathog Glob Health* 2015; 109: 309-318.

[8] Rebelo Gomes E, Ribeiro-Vaz I, Santos CC, et al. Adverse drug reactions in adolescents: a review of reporting to a national pharmacovigilance system. *Expert Opin Drug Saf* 2020; 19: 915-922.

[9] European Parliament. *DIRECTIVE 2010/84/EU*, https://eur-lex.europa.eu/LexUriServ/LexUriServ.do?uri=OJ:L:2010:348:0074:0099:EN:PDF (2010, accessed 12 November 2020).

[10] Shamna M, Dilip C, Ajmal M, et al. A prospective study on Adverse Drug Reactions of antibiotics in a tertiary care hospital. *Saudi Pharm J* 2014; 22: 303-308.

[11] Kiguba R, Karamagi C, Bird SM. Antibiotic-associated suspected adverse drug reactions among hospitalized patients in Uganda: a prospective cohort study. *Pharmacol Res Perspect* 2017; 5: e00298.

[12] Pitts PJ, Louet H Le, Moride Y, et al. 21st century pharmacovigilance: efforts, roles, and responsibilities. *Lancet Oncol* 2016; 17: e486–e492.

[13] Centers for Disease Control and Prevention. Antibiotic Use Questions and Answers, https://www.cdc.gov/antibiotic-use/community/about/should-know.html (accessed 27 October 2020).

[14] Nicolaou KC, Chen JS, Edmonds DJ, et al. Recent Advances in the Chemistry and Biology of Naturally Occurring Antibiotics. *Angew Chemie Int Ed* 2009; 48: 660-719.

[15] Aminov RI. A Brief History of the Antibiotic Era: Lessons Learned and Challenges for the Future. *Front Microbiol*; 1. Epub ahead of print 2010. DOI: 10.3389/fmicb.2010.00134.

[16] Ribeiro da Cunha, Fonseca, Calado. Antibiotic Discovery: Where Have We Come from, Where Do We Go? *Antibiotics* 2019; 8: 45.

[17] Antibacterials for Systemic Use, https://www.whocc.no/atc_ddd_index/?code=J01&showdescription=no (accessed 27 October 2020).

[18] Wald-Dickler N, Holtom P, Spellberg B. Busting the Myth of "Static vs Cidal": A Systemic Literature Review. *Clin Infect Dis* 2018; 66: 1470-1474.

[19] Ventola CL. The antibiotic resistance crisis: part 1: causes and threats. *P T* 2015; 40: 277-83.

[20] North J. *Challenges to Tackling Antimicrobial Resistance*. Cambridge University Press. Epub ahead of print 30 April 2020. DOI: 10.1017/9781108864121.

[21] Munita JM, Arias CA. Mechanisms of Antibiotic Resistance. *Microbiol Spectr*; 4. Epub ahead of print 1 April 2016. DOI: 10.1128/microbiolspec.VMBF-0016-2015.

[22] European Centre for Disease Prevention and Control. *Antimicrobial consumption in the EU/EEA, annual epidemiological report for 2019*. Stockholm, https://www.ecdc.europa.eu/en/publications-data/surveillance-antimicrobial-consumption-europe-2019 (2020).

[23] Yam ELY, Hsu LY, Yap EP-H, et al. Antimicrobial Resistance in the Asia Pacific region: a meeting report. *Antimicrob Resist Infect Control* 2019; 8: 202.

[24] WHO. *WHO report on surveillance of antibiotic consumption: 2016-2018 early implementation*. Geneva: World Health Organization, https://www.who.int/medicines/areas/rational_use/oms-amr-amc-report-2016-2018/en/ (2018).

[25] CDC. *Antibiotic resistance threats in the United States, 2019*. Atlanta, GA: U.S. Department of Health and Human Services, CDC. Epub ahead of print November 2019. DOI: 10.15620/cdc:82532.

[26] CDC. *Antibiotic Use in the United States, 2018 Update: Progress and Opportunities*. Atlanta, GA: U.S. Department of Health and Human Services, CDC, https://www.cdc.gov/antibiotic-use/stewardship-report/pdf/stewardship-report-2018-508.pdf (2019).

[27] Nahrgang, Saskia; Nolte, Ellen; Rechel B. Antimicrobial Resistance. In: *The role of public health organizations in addressing public health problems in Europe*. Copenhagen, Denmark: European Observatory on Health Systems and Policies, https://www.ncbi.nlm.nih.gov/books/NBK536193/ (2018).

[28] World Health Organization. One Health, https://www.who.int/features/qa/one-health/en/ (2017).

[29] World Health Organization. *Global action plan on antimicrobial resistance*, https://www.amcra.be/swfiles/files/WHO actieplan_90.pdf (2015).

[30] Centers for Disease Control and Prevention. One Health, https://www.cdc.gov/onehealth/ (2020).

[31] European Commision. *A European One Health Action Plan against Antimicrobial Resistance*, https://ec.europa.eu/health/sites/health/files/antimicrobial_resistance/docs/amr_2017_action-plan.pdf (2017).

[32] Roque F, Teixeira-Rodrigues A, Breitenfeld L, et al. Decreasing antibiotic use through a joint intervention targeting physicians and pharmacists. *Future Microbiol* 2016; 11: 877-886.

[33] Teixeira Rodrigues A, Roque F, Piñeiro-Lamas M, et al. Effectiveness of an intervention to improve antibiotic-prescribing behaviour in primary care: a controlled, interrupted time-series study. *J Antimicrob Chemother* 2019; 74: 2788-2796.

[34] Teixeira Rodrigues A, Ferreira M, Roque F, et al. Physicians' attitudes and knowledge concerning antibiotic prescription and resistance: questionnaire development and reliability. *BMC Infect Dis* 2015; 16: 7.

[35] Oliveira I, Rego C, Semedo G, et al. Systematic Review on the Impact of

Guidelines Adherence on Antibiotic Prescription in Respiratory Infections. *Antibiotics* 2020; 9: 546.

[36] Beninger P. Pharmacovigilance: An Overview. *Clin Ther* 2018; 40: 1991-2004.

[37] Coleman JJ, Pontefract SK. Adverse drug reactions. *Clin Med (Northfield Il)* 2016; 16: 481-485.

[38] Baldo P, Francescon S, Fornasier G. Pharmacovigilance workflow in Europe and Italy and pharmacovigilance terminology. *Int J Clin Pharm* 2018; 40: 748-753.

[39] European Medicines Agency. *Guideline on good pharmacovigilance practices (GVP) Module VI – Collection, management and submission of reports of suspected adverse reactions to medicinal products*, https://www.ema.europa.eu/en/documents/regulatory-procedural-guideline/guideline-good-pharmacovigilance-practices-gvp-module-vi-collection-management-submission-reports_en.pdf (2017).

[40] Edwards IR, Aronson JK. Adverse drug reactions: definitions, diagnosis, and management. *Lancet* 2000; 356: 1255-1259.

[41] Aronson JK. Joining the DoTS: new approach to classifying adverse drug reactions. *BMJ* 2003; 327: 1222-1225.

[42] Laporte J-R. Fifty years of pharmacovigilance - Medicines safety and public health. *Pharmacoepidemiol Drug Saf* 2016; 25: 725-732.

[43] Bouvy JC, De Bruin ML, Koopmanschap MA. Epidemiology of Adverse Drug Reactions in Europe: A Review of Recent Observational Studies. *Drug Saf* 2015; 38: 437-453.

[44] Akhideno P, Fasipe O, Isah A, et al. Pattern of medications causing adverse drug reactions and the predisposing risk factors among medical in-patients in clinical practice: A prospective study. *J Med Sci* 2019; 39: 18.

[45] Tamma PD, Avdic E, Li DX, et al. Association of Adverse Events With Antibiotic Use in Hospitalized Patients. *JAMA Intern Med* 2017; 177: 1308.

[46] Aronson JK. *Meyler's Side Effects of Drugs - The International Encyclopedia of Adverse Drug Reactions and Interactions*. 16th ed. Elsevier Science, 2015.

[47] Postigo R, Brosch S, Slattery J, et al. EudraVigilance Medicines Safety Database: Publicly Accessible Data for Research and Public Health Protection. *Drug Saf* 2018; 41: 665-675.

[48] System of Information and Monitoring of the Portuguese National Health System. SIM@SNS, https://bicsp.min-saude.pt/pt/investigacao/Paginas/medicamentoprescritor_publico.aspx?isdlg=1 (accessed 12 November 2020).

[49] Serviços Partilhados do Ministério da Saúde (SPMS). Bilhete de Identidade dos Cuidados de Saúde Primários, https://bicsp.min-saude.pt/pt/investigacao/Paginas/medicamentoprescritor_publico.aspx?isdlg=1 (accessed 11 November 2020).

[50] Center UM. VigiBase, http://www.vigiaccess.org/.

[51] EMA. EudraVigilance, http://www.adrreports.eu/en/index.html (accessed 12 November 2020).

[52] Bhattacharya S. The facts about penicillin allergy: a review. *J Adv Pharm Technol Res* 2010; 1: 11-7.

[53] Nogueira Guerra L, Herdeiro MT, Ribeiro-Vaz I, et al. Adverse drug reactions in children: a ten-year review of reporting to the Portuguese Pharmacovigilance System. *Expert Opin Drug Saf* 2015; 14: 1805-1813.

[54] Principi N, Esposito S. Antibiotic-related adverse events in paediatrics: unique characteristics. *Expert Opin Drug Saf* 2019; 18: 795-802.

[55] Smyth RMD, Gargon E, Kirkham J, et al. Adverse Drug Reactions in Children—A Systematic Review. *PLoS One* 2012; 7: e24061.

[56] Lovegrove MC, Geller AI, Fleming-Dutra KE, et al. US Emergency Department Visits for Adverse Drug Events From Antibiotics in Children, 2011-2015. *J Pediatric Infect Dis Soc* 2019; 8: 384-391.

[57] Bookstaver PB, Bland CM, Griffin B, et al. A Review of Antibiotic Use in Pregnancy. *Pharmacother J Hum Pharmacol Drug Ther* 2015; 35: 1052-1062.

[58] Kuperman AA, Koren O. Antibiotic use during pregnancy: how bad is it? *BMC Med* 2016; 14: 91.

[59] Fan H, Gilbert R, O'Callaghan F, et al. Associations between macrolide antibiotics prescribing during pregnancy and adverse child outcomes in the UK: population based cohort study. *BMJ* 2020; m331.

[60] Davies EA, O'Mahony MS. Adverse drug reactions in special populations - the elderly. *Br J Clin Pharmacol* 2015; 80: 796-807.

[61] Giarratano A, Green S EL, Nicolau DP. Review of antimicrobial use and considerations in the elderly population. *Clin Interv Aging* 2018; Volume 13: 657-667.

Chapter 5

Evaluation of the Medication Safety of Chemotherapy Drugs

Sayna Jabalpeikar

Abstract

To evaluate the medication safety of chemotherapy drugs at a tertiary care hospital, with complete reporting of prescription errors, classifying prescription errors, complete detailing of watched medication administration errors (MAEs) by nurses, ordering watched MAEs, and figuring improvement methodologies. Likewise, in relation to side effects, how to overcome side effects, which antiemetic treatments to use, how to survey the appropriateness of requesting and apportioning. An imminent, observational, non-interventional contemplate study was driven at the Oncology Department, Baptist Hospital, Bangalore for half a year. All the data was collected from patient medical records according to case record structure. An aggregate of 70 patients tolerating chemotherapy were observed for information on a sort of side effects, prescription missteps and other relevant information like demographic findings, treatments, and drugs used to manage the adverse effects (AEs) collected from the patient's medical records. The data was characterized reliant on various parameters. The watched side effects according to different organ frameworks were orchestrated and appeared differently in relation to the distributed writing and bundle embeds. Among the 70 patients, 22 (31.4%) were males and 48 (68.57%) were females. Moreover, the age interval within these two groups was of 20–65. From the 70 patients, the number of chemotherapy cycles was of one for 14 (20%) patients, two for 16 (22.85%), three for 16 (22.85%), four for 5 (7.14%), five for 6 (8.57%), six for 9 (12.85%), and more than six for 4 (5.71%) patients, mostly due to maintenance chemotherapy. The evaluation of our information uncovered that the cancer with the most elevated predominance was breast cancer (24.28%), pursued by blood and bone marrow cancer (5.71%) in females, whereas in males were blood and bone marrow (4.28%), followed by lung cancer (2.85%), non-Hodgkin lymphoma (2.85%), and colon cancer (2.85%). The present study demonstrated that in both gender groups, the most influenced organ framework was gastro intestinal tract (GIT), trailed by skin and subcutaneous tissue, musculoskeletal, blood and nervous system. The most prescribed antiemetic drug was ondansetron (81.42%), and the normally endorsed chemotherapy agents in our setting were shown to be cisplatin (21.42%), carboplatin (17.14%), and paclitaxel (14.28%). The total percentage of errors on the 70 prescriptions was 24.28. Most of the errors were due to drug–drug interactions (10%). The total percentage of errors in drug administration performed by nurses was found to be 11.42%, out of which in 2.85% of the cases, it was used the wrong drug dose. The adverse impacts related with the usage of anticancer medication were surveyed for half a year. The AEs most commonly experienced suggest that for all intents and purposes, all the patients accepting cytotoxic drugs suffered at least one AE. The critical announced MAE rates on our hospital ward (0.04% of medication administration and 0.03% MAE/patient admission) send out an impression of being generally low due to the utilization of current security rules. Emphasize on deep understanding of MAE at individual foundations, is likely going to result in important procedure changes, improved effectiveness of MAE detailing, and various focal points.

Keywords: medication safety, chemotherapy drugs, adverse effects, side effects, error in prescription, error in administration, emetogenic chemotherapy, antiemetic drugs, and comparison of antiemetic guidelines

1. Introduction

Medication safety has been recognized to be important in the provision of patient care for a long time. With the evidence pointing to medication errors (MEs) as one of the leading causes of avoidable complications and deaths, there is a pressing need for a better understanding of the nature and scope of MEs, and the will to improve the current clinical delivery systems. [1]

The chemotherapeutic agents are associated with severe adverse effects (AEs), leading to economic burden and decreased quality of life. [2]

The issue of medication safety in chemotherapy drugs is highly significant when anticancer therapy is used as a treatment modality due to the high hazards derived from these agents and the disease context in which they are used. [2]

The purpose of this chapter is to determine the error rate in prescribing, dispensing and administration of chemotherapy drugs and related agents used in the treatment of cancer, and to promote the prevention of MEs to improve patient safety.

The complexity of treatment regimens designed to achieve the maximal anti-cancer effect balanced against acceptable toxicity leaves limited margin for error. Overdosing can result in death due to treatment associated AEs, while under dosing can have significant implications for the management of the disease and to the patient outcome. [3]

MEs can occur for a number of reasons. Errors can occur when human and system factors interact with the complex process of prescribing, dispensing and administration drugs, to produce an unintended and potentially harmful outcome.

With an extreme move in the comprehension of medical errors through the production of the 1999 Institute of Medicine (IOM) report, To Err is Human, [4], the IOM board required a change in the manner health-care experts comprehend therapeutic error by standards ranging from subjective psychology to human factors, and investigation of human execution in workplaces.

The enhancements in aeronautics and other security-arranged businesses, for instance, chemical engineering, manufacturing, and nuclear power, showed that complex systems, instead of individual specialists, were the fundamental wellsprings of error and thus an objective for improvement openings through modifications, systematization, and innovation. Sentinel events in oncology, including the death of Betsy Lehman in 1994 at Boston's Dana-Farber Cancer Institute, conspicuously highlighted the open impression of medicinal error. Past research has seemed certain patients are at an extended danger of preventable damage, which is associated with their restricted Physiological Reserve, (physiological reserve is the capacity of an organ or body part to fulfill its physiological activity), which typically joins patients with intense ailments, comorbidities, different prescriptions, and harmful sickness. [5, 6]

Chemotherapeutic prescriptions have a constrained therapeutic index and the dosage expected to give an effective response is conventionally poisonous to the body's quickly multiplying cells. The typical tissues antagonistically affected by the chemotherapy drugs are those, which are rapidly partitioning, like bone marrow, gastrointestinal tract and hair follicles. Chemotherapy drugs also have other organ explicit toxicities. Moreover, a couple of drugs that are usually associated with speedy adverse reactions are a consequence of their biochemical nature, rather than their activity against tumors. The use of some cancer chemotherapy drugs have been associated with a few AEs, usually going from mild nausea to fatal myelosuppression. [7]

During the most recent decade, various examinations have shown that medication inducing morbidity and mortality is one of the most significant general medical issues. [8]

Clinicians should be aware that chemotherapy induced nausea and vomiting (CINV) is one of the most complicated side effects of chemotherapy. With the correct use of antiemetics, CINV can be prevented in almost 70% up to 80% of the patients. [9]

The goal of each antiemetic treatment is to abrogate nausea and vomiting. Twenty years back, nausea and vomiting were typical AEs resulting from specific sorts of chemotherapy and which obliged up to 20% of the patients to postpone or decay possibly corrective treatments [10]. Clinical and major research over the span of ongoing years has provoked persistent enhancements in the control of CINV. [11]

The improvement of the serotonin receptor antagonists (5-HT3RAs) in the mid-1990s was a standout among the most imperative advances in the chemotherapy of cancer patients. [12, 13] Another group of antiemetics discovered, the neurokinin1-receptor antagonist (NK1RA), and the essential medication in this class, aprepitant, were consolidated into the refreshed antiemetic rules. [14, 15]

In 1998, the main Multinational Association of Supportive Care in Cancer (MASCC) antiemetic rules reliant on the outcomes of the Perugia understanding, were brought together and were distributed worldwide, trailed by the American Society of Clinical Oncology (ASCO) rules in 1999 [16]. The two guidelines, similarly as the National Comprehensive Cancer Network (NCCN) rules, invigorated [17, 18]. The audit of antiemetics, contrasts these three rules, regarding the utilization of antiemetics in chemotherapy settings.

2. Medication error rate

The ME rate was dictated by ascertaining the level of errors. The numerators in the proportion, is the absolute number of error. The numerator in the proportion is the complete number of error that they watch, the denominator is called "opportunities for errors" and incorporates every single watched dosage that is controlled, in addition to the portions requested but not directed. [19, 20]

$$\text{Medication error rate} = \frac{\text{Number of errors observed}}{\text{Opportunities for errors}} * 100 \tag{1}$$

Endorsing error happens at the time a prescriber orders a medication for a particular patient. The error might be due to dosage form, number of dosages, dose structure, course of association, and length of treatment. The MEs, including cancer chemotherapeutic administrators, may be particularly unsafe as these drugs have a limited helpful profile for which prescriptions have a confined association that may result in expanded toxicity and/or decreased tumor response. Furthermore, antineoplastic administrators are consistently coordinated to be applied to more established patients with comorbidities and it is novel and complex treatment for nurses and medication assistants. Along these lines, antineoplastic masters are among the most outstanding reasons of ME. [1, 19, 20]

3. Theoretical framework

According to a study on MEs on a Community Hospital Oncology Ward, it was found that out of 141 medication administration errors (MAEs) detected amid the study period, the most persistent ones were administration errors, 41%, while 38% were either nurse or pharmacy dispensing errors, and 21% constituted order writing and transcribing errors. Out of these MAEs, only three errors resulted from adverse drug events. [20]

In another study based on the AEs.of.anticancer.drugs.in.an Oncology Centre of a Tertiary Care Hospital, from a total of 130 evaluated cases, 60 cases comprised males (46.2%), and 70 comprised females (53.8%). The most prevalent cancers among females were breast cancer and cervical cancer, whereas lung cancer and urinary bladder cancer were the most common among males. Nausea (48.5%), decreased appetite (39.2%), alopecia (37.7%), anemia (35.4%), vomiting (31.5%), and nail discoloration (30%) were the most frequently reported AEs. The commonly used pre medication were ondansetron, dexamethasone, aprepitant and proton pump inhibitors, individually or in combination. [21]

Moreover, a study regarding side effects of chemotherapy among cancer patients revealed that out of 99 patients, the majority had their age between 45–64 years (73.3%) and were females (93.3%). Nausea and vomiting were two of the most common side effects (83.3% and 78.9% respectively) reported.

Other common side effects were hair loss and loss of appetite. Also 6.7% of patients experienced peripheral neuropathy symptoms. [22]

3.1 Chemotherapy-induced emesis

With respect to the emetogenicity potential, the chemotherapy agents can be classified into four emetic risk groups: [23].

High (≥90% of patients experienced nausea and vomiting when no prophylactic antiemetic protection was provided);

Moderate (30–90% of patients experienced nausea and vomiting when no prophylactic antiemetic protection was provided);

Low (10–30% of patients experienced nausea and vomiting when no prophylactic antiemetic protection was provided);

Minimal (≤10% of patients, experienced nausea and vomiting when no prophylactic antiemetic protection was provided), as suggested by all three guidelines. [17, 18, 23, 24]. Hence, antiemetic prophylaxis is directly proportional to the emetogenic potential of the chemotherapy.

The emetogenic potential of the drugs is different in each guideline. In the MASCC guideline in particular, the emetogenic potential of oral chemotherapeutic agents is different from intravenous chemotherapeutic agents. In MASCC and NCCN guidelines, intravenous etoposide is labeled as having low emetogenic potential. However, oral etoposide is usually classified as having moderate emetogenic potential, implying that there is a 30%–90% incidence of emesis [24].

In a recently published study by Einhorn *et al*, [25] oral etoposide indeed seemed to have only low emetogenic potential. Additionally, althought imatinib is classified by the MASCC and NCCN guidelines as a moderate emetogenic agent, the daily use of antiemetics is not recommended in the special case of imatinib by the NCCN.

The ASCO guidelines do not implicate any of the oral chemotherapeutic agents in their classification system [23].

3.2 Patient-related risk factors inducing emesis

Patient-related risk factors, including age (young age usually experience more nausea and vomiting), gender (females generally experience more nausea and vomiting compared to males), a history of alcohol intake, a history of an emesis experience amid pregnancy, impaired quality of life, and also a history of previous chemotherapy, are known to increase the risk for CINV. [23, 26, 27]

3.3 Antiemetic agents

3.3.1 5-hydroxytryptamine receptor antagonists (5-HT3RAs)

These are the most effective antiemetic agents in the prophylaxis of acute CINV. [28]

The different 5-HT3RAs, namely dolasetron, granisetron, ondansetron, palonosetron and, tropisetron appear to be interchangeable. The lowest fully effective single dose for each agent should be use. The oral and intravenous routes are similarly effective. These statements are supported by all three guidelines. [29]

1. **Dolasetron:** All three guidelines recommend the same doses of dolasetron, which are 100 mg or 1.8 mg/kg intravenously, and 100 mg orally. [29]

2. **Granisetron:** All three guidelines recommend granisetron at a dose of 1 mg or 0.01 mg/kg intravenously, and 2 mg orally (MASCC and ASCO) or 1–2 mg orally (NCCN). [29, 30]

3. **Ondansetron:** with respect to the dosing of ondansetron, different statements are given. For example, the NCCN guidelines recommend ondansetron at a dose of 16–24 mg orally and 8–12 mg (maximum, 32 mg) intravenously, whereas the MASCC and ASCO guidelines recommend ondansetron at a dose of 24 mg orally (MASCC, 16 mg orally for moderately emetogenic chemotherapy) and 8 mg or 0.15 mg/kg I.V. In a recently published meta-analysis comparing low-dose ondansetron (8 mg) with high-dose ondansetron (24 or 32 mg), in a sub analysis in cisplatin based chemotherapy, high-dose ondansetron appeared to be more effective [29].

4. **Palonosetron:** All three guidelines recommend palonosetron at a dose of 0.25 mg intravenously. Oral palonosetron is not yet available. Palonosetron has a significantly longer half-life and a higher binding activity compared to the other 5-HT3RA. The actual role of palonosetron in comparison with the other available 5-HT3RA has been controversially discussed in the guidelines. However, none of the three guidelines designates a preferred 5-HT3RA, although palonosetron outperformed ondansetron and dolasetron in some secondary endpoints in one reported study. [29, 31]. For a better understanding, the results of the three available randomized studies with palonosetron in the acute phase are outlined, where it was found that palnosetron's effect was significantly superior to ondansetron. [29, 31, 32].

5. **Tropisetron:** An orally or intravenously dose of 5 mg is recommended for tropisetron according to the ASCO and MASCC guidelines. [29]

3.3.2 Steroids

Steroids are commonly used in the treatment of several cancers, such as lymphoma and leukemia as they help to destroy cancer cells and render chemotherapy more effective reduce allergy reaction to certain drugs, and also protect the patient from having nausea and vomiting after a round of chemotherapy. Steroids used in chemotherapy include prednisolone, methyl prednisolone, and dexamethasone. [33, 34]

Dexamethasone: Although not approved as an antiemetic, dexamethasone plays a major role in the prevention of acute and delayed CINV and is an integral component of almost all antiemetic regimens [33, 34].All three guidelines recommend the use of dexamethasone for the acute prevention of highly, moderately, and low emetogenic chemotherapy.

According to the three guidelines, for the prevention of delayed emesis, dexamethasone is recommended in combination with aprepitant for highly emetogenic chemotherapy (MASCC, ASCO, NCCN), but not for moderately emetogenic chemotherapy (MASCC, ASCO). Only the NCCN guidelines suggest dexamethasone as a possible combination partner for aprepitant with moderately emetogenic chemotherapy.

This recommendation of the MASCC and ASCO expert panel is mostly drive by the study of Warr *et al.* [35] in patients receiving moderately emetogenic chemotherapy. In this study, aprepitant is given as monotherapy for the prevention of delayed CINV, and a complete response rate of 55%, in comparison with 49% for ondansetron, was achieved in the delayed phase.

This result might suggest that the combination of dexamethasone and aprepitant in the delayed phase would have greater antiemetic efficacy. Thus this might be the reason why the NCCN panel was recommending this combination in the moderately emetogenic setting in the delayed phase.

Further studies are warranted to clarify this clinically important question. When combined with aprepitant, dose reduction of dexamethasone (dexamethasone is a sensitive substrate of the cytochrome P450 [CYP450] 3A4 enzyme) has to be undertaken. For the prevention of acute CINV, the dose of choice should be 20 mg of dexamethasone (12 mg when co administered with aprepitant). For highly emetogenic chemotherapy a single dose of 8 mg dexamethasone (12 mg in the NCCN guidelines) is enough. For moderately emetogenic chemotherapy, these dose recommendations were largely driven by studies from the Italian Group for Antiemetic Research [36, 37].

3.3.3 Neurokinin 1 receptor antagonists (NK1RAs)

NK1 receptor antagonists are in a class of drugs used to treat nausea and vomiting associated with chemotherapy. Aprepitant, casopitant, fosaprepitant, and rolapitant are some examples of NK1 drugs.

Aprepitant: Is the first representative of this new group that blocks the NK1 receptor in the brainstem emetic center and gastrointestinal tract [38]. So far, it is only available for oral use and should be administered as 125 mg on day one, and 80 mg on day two and day three as recommended by all three guidelines. Published studies have shown that the addition of NK1RAs to standard antiemetic therapy (5HT3RA plus dexamethasone) appears to have a significant effect in controlling cisplatin-induced acute as well as delayed emesis.

In all studies the aprepitant regimen was more pronounced in the delayed phase of CINV [38–40]. The use of aprepitant is suggested for both highly and moderately emetogenic chemotherapy by all three guidelines.

In the moderately emetogenic setting, one study has been published and, formed the basis for the recommendation of aprepitant for anthracycline and cyclophosphamide– based emetogenic chemotherapy. In this study [35], the triple combination of ondansetron, dexamethasone, and aprepitant used in the first 24 hours, followed by aprepitant monotherapy for another 2 days, proved to be superior to the whole 5-day study period (51% *vs* 42%). However, no significant differences were observed in the delayed period (49% *vs* 55%), possibly because only patients receiving an anthracycline and cyclophosphamide– based regimen were included in this study.

The MASCC and ASCO guidelines restricted the recommendation of the triple combination in the moderately emetogenic setting due to this "high-risk" chemotherapeutic regimen.

The NCCN guidelines, however, recommended aprepitant in the moderately emetogenic setting in selected patients based on the emetogenic potential of the chemotherapy.

In the MASCC guidelines, it was noted that no trials have compared so far, the combination of aprepitant with dexamethasone for delayed emesis with the previous standard of dexamethasone combined with a 5-HT3RA in highly emetogenic chemotherapy. [16] In the meantime, a study addressing this question [40] showed that the effect obtained from the combination of aprepitant with dexamethasone was superior to one resulting from the combination of ondansetron and dexamethasone in the delayed phase.

Aprepitant is a moderate inhibitor of CYP3A4; therefore, the dexamethasone dose has to be reduced, as discussed before. Theoretical concerns that aprepitant might interact with chemotherapeutic agents could not be demonstrated in preclinical and clinical studies so far [16, 40, 41].

3.3.4 Metoclopramide

Metoclopramide was part of the former MASCC, ASCO, and NCCN guidelines and was suggested for the prevention of delayed emesis [16, 20]. Although metoclopramide has proved to be as effective as 5-HT3RA when combined with steroids in the prevention of delayed CINV [42, 43] it is not recommended in the new guidelines in this setting. However, because 5-HT3RAs are recommended as an alternative to dexamethasone in the delayed phase for moderately emetogenic chemotherapy, metoclopramide might also be an adequate alternative, although not recommended by the guidelines.

3.3.5 Cannabinoids

The MASCC guidelines state that cannabinoids can be considered for refractory nausea and vomiting and as a rescue antiemetic. However, due to the weak antiemetic efficacy with potentially high side effects including, sedation, euphoria, dysphoria, dizziness, and hallucination, cannabinoids are not recommended as first-line treatment for the prevention of CINV.

In the ASCO and NCCN guidelines, cannabinoids are advised in patients intolerant or refractory to 5-HT3RAs or steroids and aprepitant.

Interestingly, a systematic review addressing the efficacy of oral cannabinoids in the prevention of nausea and vomiting revealed, that cannabinoids were slightly more efficient than conventional anti emetics (e.g., metoclopramide, phenothiazines, haloperidol.). However, their usefulness was generally limited by the high incidence of toxic effects, such as dizziness, dysphoria, and hallucinations. [44–46]

3.3.6 Benzodiazepines

Benzodiazepines can be useful in controlling anxiety and reduction of anticipatory CINV or in patients with refractory and breakthrough emesis, as suggested by all three guidelines. [47]

3.3.7 Antihistamines

The most common antihistamines used are diphenhydramine and hydroxyzine. Nevertheless, the available studies have not shown any significant antiemetic activity in these agents. [48]

3.3.8 Olanzapine

Olanzapine is an atypical antipsychotic drug with, antiemetic potential due to its action at multiple receptor sites implicated in the control of nausea and vomiting. [49] In a phase II trial where olanzapine was used in combination with granisetron and dexamethasone for the prevention of CINV, the combination therapy proved to be highly effective in controlling acute and delayed CINV in patients receiving highly and moderately emetogenic chemotherapy. [50] The latest phase II study published by Navari *et al*. [51] showed exceptionally high complete protection rates from both acute and delayed CINV when using a combination of palonosetron (day 1), dexamethasone (day 1), and olanzapine (days 1–4) in patients receiving highly or moderately emetogenic chemotherapy. Consequently, olanzapine is mentioned by the MASCC and NCCN guidelines for the treatment of refractory and breakthrough emesis with a suggested dose of 2.5–5 mg.

3.4 Classification of CINV based on the guidelines

According to the guidelines CINV can be differentiated into five categories: [52].

1. When nausea and vomiting occur within 24 hours of initial administration of chemotherapy is known as acute onset, which is mostly due to serotonin-related agents.

2. When nausea and vomiting occur 24 hours to several days after initial treatment is known as delayed onset, which is due to substance P-related agents.

3. Anticipatory nausea and vomiting is observed in patients whose emetic episodes were triggered by taste, odor sight, thoughts, anxiety, or had a history of poor response to antiemetic agents or received inadequate antiemetic prophylaxis in the previous cycle of chemotherapy.

4. Breakthrough CINV is defined as vomiting and/or nausea that occur within five days of chemotherapy administration after the use of guideline directed prophylactic antiemetic agents. This type of CINV usually requires immediate treatment or requires "rescue" with additional antiemetics.

5. Refractory CINV is defined as vomiting and/or nausea occurring after chemotherapy, usually in subsequent chemotherapy cycles after guideline directed prophylactic antiemetic agents have failed in earlier cycles.

3.5 Prevention of CINV

3.5.1 Regimens linked to a high incidence of nausea and vomiting are referred as highly emetogenic chemotherapy (≥90%)

Acute CINV: All three guidelines suggest the combination of a 5-HT3RA, dexamethasone, and aprepitant within the first 24 hours of chemotherapy.

Delayed CINV: All three guidelines suggest the combination of dexamethasone and aprepitant for delayed CINV. Trials have indicated that from 60% to nearly 90% of patients receiving cisplatin will experience delayed emesis if not given preventive anti emetics. Therefore, appropriate prophylaxis is necessary [17, 52, 53].

3.5.2 Regimens linked to a moderate incidence of nausea and vomiting are referred as moderately emetogenic chemotherapy (30–90%)

Acute CINV: All three guidelines recommend the combination of a 5-HT3RA plus dexamethasone with or without aprepitant for acute CINV. However, the key question in this setting is whether aprepitant should be part of the antiemetic prophylaxis or not. The ASCO and MASCC guidelines recommend the triple combination (a 5HT3RA, dexamethasone, and aprepitant) for patients receiving the combination of an anthracycline and cyclophosphamide–based regimen. The NCCN guidelines, however, broadened the spectrum of the use and suggest using the triple combination in patients receiving other chemotherapy agents of moderately emetogenic risk like carboplatin, epirubicin, ifosfamide, or irinotecan [17, 52, 53].

Delayed CINV: Dexamethasone is the preferred agent to be used for delayed CINV. Nonetheless, when aprepitant is used for the prevention of acute CINV then it should also be used for the prophylaxis of delayed CINV as mono therapy, as stated by the MASCC and ASCO guidelines. As discussed before, the NCCN guidelines suggest aprepitant with or without dexamethasone in this situation. A 5-HT3RA can be used as an alternative, although their therapeutic role in the delayed phase is rather limited [34]. In contrast to all three previously published guidelines, metoclopramide is not reflected in the new guidelines as an alternative option [17, 52, 53].

3.5.3 Regimens linked to a low incidence of nausea and vomiting are referred as low emetogenic chemotherapy (10–30%)

The MASCC and ASCO guidelines in unison recommend the use of a steroid alone in the first 24 hours and no prophylaxis beyond 24 hours for acute CINV. The NCCN guidelines recommend prochlorperazine or metoclopramide as well, as alternative drugs to dexamethasone [17, 52, 53].

3.5.4 Regimens linked to a minimal incidence of nausea and vomiting are referred to as minimally emetogenic chemotherapy (≤10%)

All three guidelines suggest that, for patients treated with agents of low emetic risk, no antiemetic drugs should be routinely administered before chemotherapy [17, 52, 53].

3.5.5 Regimens linked to an incidence of nausea and vomiting in case of anticipatory, breakthrough or refractory chemotherapy

Anticipatory, breakthrough and refractory CINV:

Anticipatory CINV is mostly seen in patients with anxiety or patients who did not receive adequate antiemetic prophylaxis in the previous cycle [17, 52, 53].

Breakthrough CINV is defined as an event that happens in spite of optimal preventive treatment.

Refractory CINV is nausea and vomiting that recurs in subsequent cycles of therapy when all previous preventive and rescue treatments fail.

If optimal treatment has been given as prophylaxis, repeated dosing of the same agents is unlikely to be successful; the addition of dopamine-receptor antagonists (for instance, metoclopramide) might be useful, or the addition of other agents such as benzodiazepines or neuroleptics. Olanzapine, an atypical neuroleptic, could also be considered, as suggested by the MASCC and NCCN guidelines. [16]

3.5.6 Regimens, linked to CINV in case of receiving chemotherapy more than one day in a cycle

Multiple-Day chemotherapy: for patients receiving multiple day chemotherapy like, for instance with cisplatin, the MASCC guidelines recommend the use of a 5-HT3RA in combination with dexamethasone for acute CINV and dexamethasone alone for delayed CINV. The use of NK1RAs remains to be defined, as stated by the MASCC guidelines. However, the NCCN guidelines advise the application of aprepitant for at least the first 3 days, in analogy to highly emetogenic chemotherapy. Furthermore, the NCCN guidelines clearly mention the use of palonosetron in this setting [17, 52, 53].

4. MEs involving antineoplastic agents

MEs involving cancer chemotherapy agents may be particularly harmful as these drugs have a narrow therapeutic index for which incorrect dosing or administration may result in increased toxicity and/or decreased tumor response. In addition, antineoplastic agents are often administered to older patients with comorbidities and may be part of novel and complex treatment protocols less familiar to nurses and pharmacists. As a result, antineoplastic agents are among the most common causes of ME-related deaths. These concerns have led to an update of national guidelines, including recommendations for a systems approach consisting of multidisciplinary monitoring of medication use, prescribing guidelines, preparation and dispensing methods, and medication administration. [54]

5. Materials and methods

An imminent, observational, non-interventional study was led at the Oncology Department, Baptist Hospital, Bangalore for half a year. All patient related- data was gathered according to case record structure. During a 6 months period, I directed an imminent report on the Oncology Ward in a Tertiary Care Hospital, with the following objectives:

- Complete reporting of prescription errors
- Classify prescription errors
- Complete revealing of MAEs errors detected by nurses
- Classify watched MAEs, and
- Formulate improvement procedures.
- Monitor and register the occurrence of side effects
- Assess how to overcome side effects?
- Evaluate the antiemetic treatments used,

A survey review of a self-assertively picked test of 70 chemotherapy solicitations to assess the appropriateness of mentioning and administering was conducted. An aggregate of 70 patients getting chemotherapy met for information on sort of side effects, MEs and other pertinent relevant information like, diagnosis, treatment, drugs utilized, and arrangement with the AEs were assembled from the patient's medical records. The data was arranged reliant on various parameters.

The MAEs are described as a preventable oversight in medicine association due to error beginning in requesting, apportioning, or overseeing. It includes association of (1) wrong prescription, (2) wrong dose, (3) wrong route, (4) wrong time, (5) a medication to which the patient has a known sensitivity, as well as, (6) a prescription with multiple drugs cooperation with another prescription. The patients accepting investigation included patients with affirmed malignancies who confessed that go chemotherapy in oncology wards.

As we expect to survey the resulting side effects a 6 month examination period was arranged. The number of patients getting chemotherapy in oncology ward for a half-year time span were utilized to appraise the sample measure.

6. Results and discussion

6.1 Demographic details

Age and sex:

Among the 70 patients, 22(31.4%) were males and 48(68.57%) were females. A further order dependent on the age uncovered that in the majority of the patients, both males and females were in the age range of 20–65 years. (**Table 1**).

Number of chemotherapy cycles:

Among the 70 patients, 14(20%) had only one chemotherapy cycle. 16(22.85%) had two chemotherapy cycles, 16(22.85%) had three chemotherapy cycles, 5(7.14%) had four chemotherapy cycles, 6(8.57%) had five chemotherapy cycles, 9(12.85%) had six chemotherapy cycles and, 4(5.71%) had more than six cycles of chemotherapy, mostly due to maintenance chemotherapy.

6.2 Chemotherapy agents

The most common endorsed chemotherapy agents in our setting.were.cisplatin (21.42%), carboplatin (17.14%), paclitaxel (14.28%), oxaliplatin.(12.85%), doxorubicin.(11.42%), and docetaxel.(11.42%), as it can be observed in **Table 2** and **Figure 1**.

6.3 Clinical diagnosis of the patients

The sub-classification based on the gender, revealed that breast (24.28%), blood and bone marrow (5.71%), cervical (2.85%), ovarian (2.85%), lung (2.85), non-Hodgkin lymphoma (2.85%), colon (2.85%), stomach (2.85%), and esophageal (2.85%) cancers

Age group (years)	Number of patients	% of patients
Pediatric (0–20)	5	7.14
20–65	58	82.85
Geriatric (< 65)	7	10

Table 1.
Cancer patient's distribution according to the age groups.

Name of drug	No of prescription	% of prescription
Cisplatin	15	21.42
Carboplatin	12	17.14
Paclitaxel	10	14.28
Oxaliplatin	9	12.85
Docetaxel	8	11.42
Doxorubicin	8	11.42
Cyclophosphamide	7	10
Vincristine	5	7.14
Etoposide	4	5.71
Flurouracil	3	4.28
Ifosfamide	3	4.28
Leucovorin	3	4.28
Methotrexate	3	4.28
Zoledronic acid	3	4.28
Atgam	2	2.85
Bendamustine	2	2.85
Daunorubicin	2	2.85
Epirubicin	2	2.85
Pemetrexed	2	2.85
Vinorelbine	2	2.85
Rituximab	2	2.85
Anastrozole	1	1.42
Bleomycin	1	1.42
Bortezomib	1	1.42
Gemcitabine	1	1.42
Herceptin	1	1.42
Irinotican	1	1.42

Table 2.
Chemotherapy agents used in the setting.

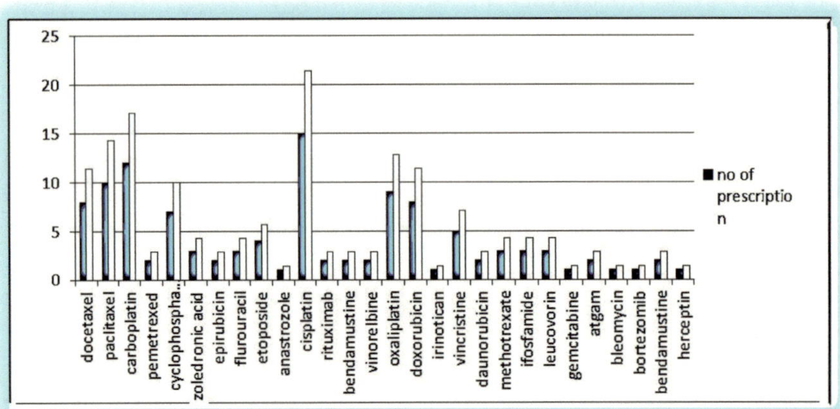

Figure 1.
Prevalence of the chemotherapy agents used in the setting according to number of prescriptions.

Type of cancer	Number of females	Number of males	% of female patients	% of male patients
anorectal	0	1	0	1.42
brain	1	0	1.42	0
breast	17	0	24.28	0
blood and bone marrow	4	3	5.71	4.28
bone	0	1	0	1.42
cervical	2	0	2.85	0
colon	2	2	2.85	2.85
esophageal	2	0	2.85	0
head and neck	1	1	1.42	1.42
Hodgkin lymphoma	1	1	1.42	1.42
larynx	0	1	0	1.42
lung	2	2	2.85	2.85
lupus	1	0	1.42	0
neck	1	0	1.42	0
non Hodgkin lymphoma	2	2	2.85	2.85
oral	1	2	1.42	2.85
ovarian	2	0	2.85	0
peritoneal	1	0	1.42	0
testicular	0	1	0	1.42
thyroid	0	1	0	1.42
tongue	0	1	0	1.42
tonsil	1	1	1.42	1.42
uterus	1	0	1.42	0
rectal	0	1	0	1.42
skin	0	1	0	1.42
muscle	1	0	1.42	0
soft tissue	1	1	1.42	1.42
stomach	2	0	2.85	0

Table 3.
Cancer prevalence among the study patients.

were the most prevalent types of cancer in females. On the other hand, blood and bone marrow (4.28%), lung (2.85%), non-Hodgkin lymphoma (2.85%), colon (2.85%), and oral (2.85%) cancers were the most prevalent in males as it can be seen in **Table 3**.

Furthermore, the most common type of cancer in the age group of 0–20 years was blood and bone marrow cancer (4.28%), while within the age group 20–65 years was breast cancer (24.28%) in females and oral cancer (2.85%) in males. In addition, in adults over 65 years breast cancer (2.85%) was the most prevalent in females. While in men there was not any significant type, as the occurrence of all the cancer types were shown to be equal (**Figure 2**).

6.4 Side effects

According to **Table 4**, the most influenced organ framework in both females and males was gastro intestinal tract (GIT), trailed by skin and subcutaneous tissue, musculoskeletal, blood, and nervous systems. Most of the patients have suffered the side

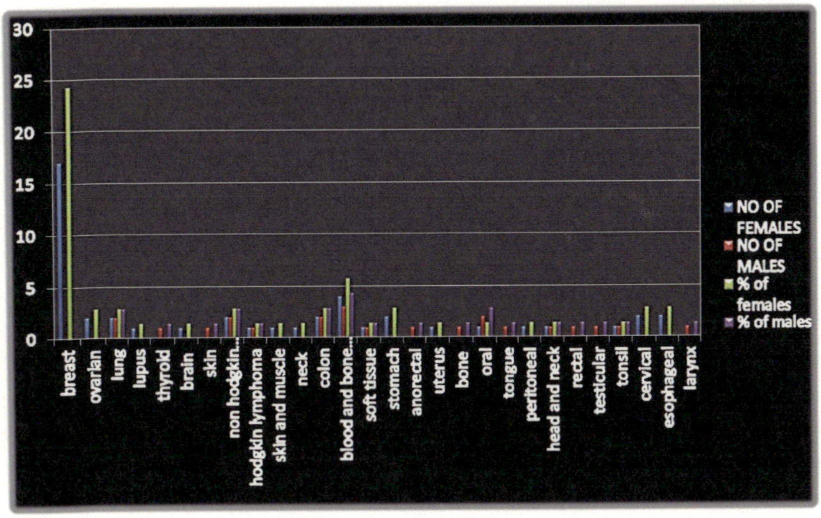

Figure 2.
Cancer prevalence among the study patients according to gender.

Organ system	side effect	Number of patients	% of patients
ALLERGIC REACTIONS	Anaphylaxis	4	5.71
	Hot flashes	1	1.42
	Itching	2	2.85
	Rash	3	4.28
	Redness	4	5.71
	Serum sickness like syndrome	2	2.85
	Swelling	5	7.14
ASTHENIA (weakness) AND CHRONIC PAIN	Fatigue	2	2.85
	Feeling weak or tired	19	27.14
	Fibromyalgia (pain all over the body)	43	61.42
BLOOD AND LYMPHATIC DISORDERS	Anemia	14	20
	Bleeding	20	28.57
	Bone marrow depression (myeloid suppression)	3	4.28
	Hemolysis	2	2.85
	Leukopenia	5	7.14
	Risk of infection	16	22.85
	Thrombocytopenia (low platelet count)	4	5.71

Organ system	side effect	Number of patients	% of patients
GIT DISORDERS	Abdominal pain	17	24.28
	Constipation	17	24.28
	Decreased appetite	32	45.71
	Diarrhea	52	74.28
	Nausea	62	88.57
	Vomiting	65	92.85
HEART AND BLOOD VESSELS DISORDERS	Chest pain	1	1.42
	Low blood pressure	16	22.85
HORMONAL DIORDERS	Missed menstrual period	3	4.28
INFECTIONS	Anal ulceration	1	1.42
	Chills	6	8.57
	Fever	7	10
	Sore eye	1	1.42
	Sore mouth	15	21.42
	Chronic wound (a wound that will not heal)	3	4.28
LIVER DISORDERS	Hepatic dysfunction	2	2.85
METABOLISM AND NUTRITIONAL DISORDERS	Anorexia	2	2.85
	Loss of taste	12	17.14
MUSCULO SKELETAL & CONNECTIVE TISSUE DISORDERS	Joint pain	17	24.28
	Muscle pain	9	12.85
NERVOUS SYSTEM DISORDERS	Dizziness	2	2.85
	Headache	2	2.85
	Insomnia	2	2.85
	Neuropathy	15	21.42
PULMONARY DISORDERS	Respiratory distress	4	5.71
RENAL &URINARY DISORDERS	Bladder irritation	2	2.85
	Blood in urine	7	10
SKIN & SUBCUTANEOUS TISSUE DISORDERS	Alopecia (hair loss)	25	35.71
	Bruising	18	25.71
	Change in skin color	3	4.28
	Nail discoloration	15	21.42
	Sweating	1	1.42

Table 4.
Side-effects prevalence and distribution depending on the organ system.

effects related to GIT, such as nausea, vomiting, diarrhea and decreased appetite. The majority of the patients experienced pain all over the body, especially in the muscle and joints and most of the patients experienced alopecia (temporary hair loss).

There are many side effects resulting from the use of chemotherapeutic agents, and rapidly developing cells have been shown to be highly affected by these agents. Hair follicles, skin, and the cells that line the GIT are some examples of the fastest growing cells in the human body, and therefore are more sensitive to the effects of chemotherapy. For this reason patients may experience hair loss, rashes, and diarrhea, respectively.

6.5 Antiemetics

6.5.1 Antiemetic therapy

Our analysis showed that all of the patients have used anti emetics in their treatment. The antiemetic used, was either a single anti emetic or a combination of antiemetics. Ondansetron was prescribed for 81.42% of the patients and used at doses of 8 mg and 16 mg, of which 8 mg was most commonly prescribed in patients recommended with a single antiemetic treatment, while the utilization of 16 mg was applied in medications containing more than one antiemetic. Dexamethasone was endorsed in 44.28% of the patients with a range of 4mg - 20 mg. Among these, 8 mg was the most normally utilized dose separately, as well as in combination with other agents. The other antiemetic, aprepitant represented 24.28% of the medications. Palonosetron was also recommended in this setting.

Aside from the antiemetics, other premedication utilized were Pantoprazole 20 mg and 40 mg, Ranitidine 150 mg and Rabeprazole 20 mg. Of these Pantoprazole, 40 mg was the most commonly used, representing 72.85% of the total prescriptions.

6.5.2 Emetogenicity and antiemetics

The utilization of more up to date antiemetic agents has profoundly diminished the occurrence of nausea and vomiting in patients receiving chemotherapy, although these symptoms were not completely forestalled. All of the patients got an antiemetic medication preceding the chemotherapy.

A 5-HT3RA like Ondansetron, Palonosetron, and a steroid drug such as dexamethasone and Aprepitant were the normally endorsed premedication in our setting, either separately or in combination. The main high hazard associated emetogenic tranquilizer used in chemotherapy in our investigation was Cisplatin. The premedication generally recommended for this setting was Ondansetron 16 mg and Dexamethasone 8 mg either separately or in combination. Cyclophosphamide, Carboplatin, Doxorubicin, Epirubicin, Oxaliplatin, Cytarabine and Ifosfamide were the drugs used in cases of moderate emetogenicity. In this study, the premedication used by the patients were Ondansetron with 8 mg and 16 mg doses, Dexamethasone with 4 mg, 8 mg, 16 mg, and 20 mg doses, Palonosetron with 0.25 mg dose and Aprepitant with 125 mg dose.

6.6 Medication errors

In this project, the error percentage in the prescription as well as in the administration of chemotherapy drugs in an oncology ward was also established.

6.6.1 Prescription error

The total error percentage reported in relation to the total number of prescriptions (70) was of 24.28%.

From these total error percentage 10% were due to drug–drug interaction, 2.8% to an unclear read, 2.8% of to lack of patient's age,2.8% to poorly written medication order, 1.42% to lack of date, and 1.4% to a bad hand writing, making it difficult to read. A complete list of errors and their associated percentage is presented in **Table 5**.

6.6.2 Administration error

Drug administration is performed by nurses. The total error percentage reported in administration of chemotherapy drugs in all the 70 patients under study was of 11.42%, out of which 2.85% were due to wrong administration dose, 2.85% to drug administration outside the guidelines, 1.42% to errors related to the speed in drug administration, and 1.45% to wrong administration technique. A complete error list is displayed in **Table 6**.

6.6.3 Prevention of medication errors

Currently, there are no sufficient strategies for estimating ME rates, and an assortment of self- reporting and non- self-reporting approaches should be utilized. The repeat of declared MEs, made the health care system to check carefully the

Type of error	Number of errors	% of errors
Wrong drugs written on prescription	0	0
Dose of drug	0	0
Dosage of drug(inappropriate or wrong dosage forms written on prescription)	0	0
Route of drug	0	0
Frequency	0	0
Date	1	1.42
Lack of patient's gender	0	0
Lack of patient's age	2	2.85
Ilegible (not clear enough to read)	2	2.85
Error in allergy documented	0	0
Error in location of treatment order	0	0
Nonstandard abbreviation used	0	0
Presence of therapeutic duplication, if any	0	0
Drug interaction if any	7	10
Food drug interaction if any	0	0
Signature of drug	0	0
Poorly written medication order	2	2.85
Miss interpreted handwritten ME	1	1.42
Fails to complete order	2	2.85
Total counts	17	24.2 8

Table 5.
Types of medication error possible to occur in drug prescription.

Type of error	No. of errors	% of errors
Wrong drugs administration by nurses	0	0
Wrong dosage administration for a recommended drugs by nurses	0	0
Failure to give a drug by the health care supplier	1	1.42
Wrong dose administration	2	2.85
Wrong administration technique	1	1.42
Drug administration to the wrong patient	0	0
Medication discontinuation failure	0	0
Omission (failure to administer an ordered dose before the next scheduled dose)	1	1.42
Double dosing by nurses	0	0
Use of incorrect (wrong)drug vehicle	0	0
Drug administration after a discontinuation order	0	0
Administration of incompatible medication	0	0
Drug administration without a physician order	0	0
Drug administration outside the established guidelines	2	2.85
Administration of an expired drug	0	0
Error in the speed of drug administration	1	1.42
Food-drug interaction	0	0
Total Counts	8	11.42

Table 6.
Types of medication errors possible to occur in drug administration.

quality with which MEs are looked for, the procedure used, the patient populace, and the importance of errors.

We have concluded that a nurse is the perfect single individual to detect a ME. Firstly, by routinely surveying the suitability of the medication and differentiating the substituted drug to the doctor-composed request. Although, the nurse may be accused of assessing the whole procedure between request composing and apportioning and afterwards, the association system.

Secondly, nurse ME declaration is the transcendent strategy in many, if not most restorative centers, give it ponder for understanding and improving the medical caretaker, revealing procedure of progressively summed up application.

Thirdly, although disliking, everyone should clearly promote a ME presentation/reduction. The ME aversion is an essential activity and a fundamental piece of significant worth in nursing. As O'Shea has noted, a nurse is accountable and responsible for the drug administration and ME anticipation is currently considered as a national nursing basic. [20]

Taking into account the jobs of drug specialists and nurses in MAE revealing cover, the benefit of including the drug store, at any foundation, would be conversely related to the adequacy of nurse reporting. Considering our decreased rate of reporting late organizations, our MAE rates are presumably similar to those detailed from different programs with compelling interception systems in place. In total, the prescribed current benchmarks displayed error rates of about 5% for association plus intercepted MEs, and roughly 0.1% to 0.2% for MAEs. These numbers appear to be commonly autonomous of patient age and chemotherapy *versus* non-chemotherapy solutions. For organization plus captured MEs, type 1 errors have been commonly typical. [a type I error is when a researcher rejects the null hypothesis that is actually true in reality. In other words, a type I error is a false positive or the conclusion that a treatment does have an effect, when in reality it does not have].

Our investigation shows that the MAE may fundamentally move toward nurse dispensing and organization. Our outcomes propose that in order to improve the formulation of MAE prevention strategies, each therapeutic center should initially be aware of where in the process of mentioning, apportioning, and overseeing medicines, the overwhelming number of MAEs starts.

6.7 Adverse effects

The overall AEs observed in both genders were practically identical. Nevertheless, the effects on gastro intestinal tract and musculoskeletal system were higher in females, which may be explained by a higher affectability of this gender by these particular effects. Iron deficiency is seen as a moderately basic condition in patients with disease, particularly those with solid tumors, lymphomas and receiving myeloid suppressive chemotherapy. Treatment for chemotherapy-induced anemia (CIA) started when the hemoglobin level fell beneath 12 mg/dl with oral or intravenous iron enhancements. Blood transfusions were picked in serious cases. In our setting, the specialists generally recommended ferrous sulfate, folic acid and Vitamin B12 prophylactic estimates, for example, great oral hygiene, avoidance of spicy food, and utilization of mild-flavored toothpaste and saline peroxide mouthwashes 3 or 4 times per day, ingrained where appropriate for limiting oral mucositis.

7. Conclusions

The AEs related with the utilization of anticancer drugs were assessed during half a year. The AE prevalence encountered and experienced suggests that all patients getting cytotoxic medication may endure at any rate one AE. Nausea, vomiting, decline appetite, alopecia, anemia, nail discoloration and anorexia were the most prevalent AEs detected. Correlation of the AEs observed with the group of individuals to achieve larger purpose did not show some new AEs. The frequency of AEs has shown to be extensively high and arouse from the utilization of existing premedication. Given the disclosures of the examination, the attempts to confine the AEs related with the anticancer medicines ought to be centered around. Expanding the mindfulness through informative intercession, actualize proper usage of premedication and non- pharmacological treatment are essential for improved personal satisfaction. Treatment rules are noteworthy in light of the fact that they outfit clinicians with a movement of proposition made from the international expert's dependent on their elucidation of the latest clinical trial data. In spite of certain qualifications among the MASCC, ASCO, and NCCN rules, all gave invigorated references and proposals to direct the perfect use of antiemetics. Nevertheless, the necessity for a progressively and reasonable usage of treatment rules is critical to improve the nature of thoughts of cancer patients. Significant detailed MAE rates on our hospital ward (0.04% of medication organizations and 0.03 MAEs/patient admission.) have all the earmarks of being generally low due to the use of current security rules. An accentuation on contemplating MAEs at individual foundations is probably going to result in significant technique changes, improved effectiveness of MAE revealing, and various other advantages.

8. Limitation

The major limitation of the study was the inability to distinguish between immediate and delayed AEs due to the difficulty of the patients in recall the AE's.

Acknowledgements

1. Karnataka College of Pharmacy, Bengaluru, India.

2. Bangalore Baptist Hospital (BBH), Bengaluru, India.

In Memory of My Grandfather Fathollah Namjoo Kerman

But grandpa's *not truly gone. Because his memory lives on. In all of us who loved him.*

Acronyms and Abbreviations

AE	Adverse effect
ASCO	American society of clinical oncology
CIA	Chemotherapy induced anemia
CINV	Chemotherapy induced nausea and vomiting
GIT	Gastro intestinal tract
IOM	Institute of medicine
MAE	Medication administration error
ME	Medication error
MASCC	Multinational association of supportive care in cancer
NCCN	National comprehensive cancer network
NK1RAs	Neurokinin 1-receptor antagonists
5-HT3RAs	Serotonin receptor antagonists

Author details

Sayna Jabalpeikar
Department of Pharmacy Practice, Karnataka College of Pharmacy,
Bengaluru, India

*Address all correspondence to: sainaj30h2@gmail.com

References

[1] Medication Safety in Hospitals: Avoiding Medication Errors in the Medication use Process 201310.4172/2167-1052.1000134Advances in Pharmacoepidemiology and Drug Safety

[2] Prevalence and significance of potential drug-drug interactions among cancer patients receiving chemotherapy 2020Mohammad Ismail, Sehrash Khan, Fahadullah Khan, Sidra Noor, Hira Sajid, Shazia Yar, Irum Rasheed10.1186/s12885-020-06855-9BMC Cancer

[3] Potential drug–drug interactions in hospitalized patients undergoing systemic chemotherapy: a prospective cohort study, 2015, Paula Stoll, Luciane Kopittke, 10.1007/s11096-015-0083-6 International Journal of Clinical Pharmacy

[4] To Err Is Human: building a safer health system Kohn L T Corrigan J M Donaldson M S Washington DC USA: Institute of Medicine/National Academy Press ISBN 0 309 06837 1

[5] Incidence of Adverse Events and Negligence in Hospitalized Patients 1991Troyen A. Brennan, Lucian L. Leape, Nan M. Laird, Liesi Hebert, A. Russell Localio, Ann G. Lawthers, Joseph P. Newhouse, Paul C. Weiler, Howard H. Hiatt10.1056/nejm199102073240604New England Journal of Medicine

[6] Quality in Australian Health Care Study 1996Ross McL Wilson, William B Runciman, Robert W Gibberd, Bernadette T Harrison, John D Hamilton10.5694/j.1326-5377.1996.tb122287.xMedical Journal of Australia

[7] Neurological adverse effects of cancer chemotherapy, 2013, Adam C.G. Thomas, 10.1097/fad.0b013e32835ed7b5 Adverse Drug Reaction Bulletin

[8] Preventing drug-related morbidity - the development of quality indicators, 2003, C. J. Morris, J. A. Cantrill, 10.1046/j.1365-2710.2003.00496.x, Journal of Clinical Pharmacy and Therapeutics

[9] Chemotherapy-Induced Nausea and Vomiting: Time for More Emphasis on Nausea? , 2015, Terry L. Ng, Brian Hutton, Mark Clemons, 10.1634/theoncologist.2014-0438, The Oncologist

[10] Global cancer statistics 2011 Ahmedin Jemal, Freddie Bray, Melissa M. Center, Jacques Ferlay, Elizabeth Ward, David Forman 10.3322/caac.20107 CA: A Cancer Journal for Clinicians.

[11] Emetogenicity of multiday chemotherapy regimens: Drug and patient factors affecting control of CINV 2009J. D. Howell, H. Brown10.1200/jco.2009.27.15_suppl.e20683Journal of Clinical Oncology

[12] Serotonin Receptor Subtypes Involved in the Elevation of Serum Corticosterone Concentration in Rats by Direct- and Indirect-Acting Serotonin Agonists, 1990, Ray W. Fuller, Harold D. Snoddy 10.1159/000125586, Neuroendocrinology

[13] How serotonin receptors regulate morphogenic signalling in neurons, 2017, Alexander Wirth, Katrin Holst, Evgeni Ponimaskin, 10.1016/j.pneurobio.2016.03.007, Progress in Neurobiology

[14] Aprepitant: novel anti-emetic brings, greater benefit for chemotherapy recipients, 2003, RM Poole, 10.2165/00128413-200314000-00029, Inpharma Weekly

[15] Aprepitant reduces nausea and vomiting after chemotherapy, 2003,

&NA, 10.2165/00128413-200313960-00032 Inpharma Weekly

[16] Prevention of chemotherapy- and radiotherapy- induced emesis: results of the 2004 Perugia International Anti-emetic Consensus Conference 200610.1093/annonc/mdj078Annals of Oncology

[17] ASCO, NCCN, MASCC/ESMO: a comparison of anti-emetic guidelines for the treatment of chemotherapy-induced nausea and vomiting in adult patients, 2018 Yasmeen Razvi, Stephanie Chan, Thomas McFarlane, Erin McKenzie, Pearl Zaki, Carlo DeAngelis, William Pidduck, Ahmad Bushehri, Edward Chow, Katarzyna Joanna Jerzak, 10.1007/s00520-018-4464-y, Supportive Care in Cancer

[18] Bridging the Critical Divide in Pain Management Guidelines From the CDC, NCCN, and ASCO for Cancer Survivors, 2018, Salimah H. Meghani, Neha Vapiwala, 10.1001/jamaoncol.2018.1574, JAMA Oncology

[19] Adverse drug events in hospitalized patients. Excess length of stay, extra costs, and attributable mortality 1997D. C. Classen10.1001/jama.277.4.301JAMA: The Journal of the American Medical Association

[20] Study of Medication Errors on a Community Hospital Oncology Ward 2006 Clyde D. Ford, Julie Killebrew, Penelope Fugitt, Janet Jacobsen, Elizabeth M. Prystas10.1200/jop.2006.2.4.149Journal of Oncology Practice

[21] A study on the adverse effects of anticancer drugs in an oncology center of a tertiary care hospital. Kirchi.c, azra afzal mounika reddy.seyed aamir ali aparna yerramilli, sanjeev sharma. International Journal of Pharmacy and Pharmaceutical Sciences. ISSN- 0975-1491 Vol 6, Suppl 2, 2014

[22] Side Effects of Chemotherapy among Cancer Patients in a Malaysian General Hospital: Experiences, Perceptions and Informational Needs from Clinical Pharmacists 2014Huan-Keat Chan, Sabrina Ismail10.7314/apjcp.2014.15.13.5305Asian Pacific Journal of Cancer Prevention

[23] Anti-emetics: American Society of Clinical Oncology Clinical Practice Guideline Update. 2017. Paul J. Hesketh, Mark G. Kris, Ethan Basch, Kari Bohlke, Sally Y. Barbour, Rebecca Anne Clark-Snow, Michael A. Danso, Kristopher Dennis, L. Lee Dupuis, Stacie B. Dusetzina, Cathy Eng, Petra C. Feyer, Karin Jordan, Kimberly Noonan, Dee Sparacio, Mark R. Somerfield, Gary H. Lyman10.1200/jco.2017.74.4789Journal of Clinical Oncology

[24] Guidelines for the control of nausea and vomiting with chemotherapy of low or minimal emetic potential Ian Olver, Rebecca A. Clark-Snow, Enzo Ballatori, Birgitte T. Espersen, Emilio Bria & Karin Jordan Supportive Care in Cancer volume 19, pages33-36(2011)

[25] Einhorn LH, Brames MJ. Emetic potential of daily oral etoposide. Support Care Cancer 2006;14:1262-1265.

[26] Evaluation of new anti-emetic agents and definition of antineoplastic agent emetogenicity—an update, 2004, Steven M. Grunberg, David Osoba, Paul J. Hesketh, Richard J. Gralla, Sussanne Borjeson, Bernardo L. Rapoport, Andreas du Bois, Maurizio Tonato 10.1007/s00520-004-0718-y, Supportive Care in Cancer

[27] Evaluation of new anti-emetic agents and definition of antineoplastic agent emetogenicity—state of the art 2010Steven M. Grunberg, David Warr, Richard J. Gralla, Bernardo L. Rapoport, Paul J. Hesketh, Karin Jordan, Birgitte T. Espersen10.1007/s00520-010-1003-xSupportive Care in Cancer

[28] Should 5-Hydroxytryptamine-3 Receptor Antagonists Be Administered Beyond 24 Hours After Chemotherapy to Prevent Delayed Emesis? Systematic Re-Evaluation of Clinical Evidence and Drug Cost Implication 2005Olga Geling, Hans-Georg Eichler10.1200/jco.2005.04.022Journal of Clinical Oncology

[29] A meta-analysis comparing the efficacy of four 5-HT3-receptor antagonists for acute chemotherapy-induced emesis 2007K. Jordan, A. Hinke, A. Grothey, W. Voigt, D. Arnold, H.-H. Wolf, H.-J. Schmoll10.1007/s00520-006-0186-7Supportive Care in Cancer

[30] Anti-emetic Efficacy of an Oral Suspension of Granisetron plus Dexamethasone and Influence of Quality of Life on Risk for Nausea and Vomiting 2005Karin Jordan, Axel Grothey, Thomas Kegel, Christian Fibich, Christoph Schöbert10.1159/000082523Oncology Research and Treatment

[31] Improved prevention of moderately emetogenic chemotherapy-induced nausea and vomiting with palonosetron, a pharmacologically novel 5-HT3 receptor antagonist 2003Peter Eisenberg, Jazmin Figueroa-Vadillo, Rosalio Zamora, Veena Charu, Julio Hajdenberg, Alan Cartmell, Alberto Macciocchi, Steven Grunberg10.1002/cncr.11817Cancer

[32] Palonosetron improves prevention of chemotherapy-induced nausea and vomiting following moderately emetogenic chemotherapy: results of a double-blind randomized phase III trial comparing single doses of palonosetron with ondansetron 2003R. Gralla, M. Lichinitser, S. Van der Vegt, H. Sleeboom, J. Mezger, C. Peschel, G. Tonini, R. Labianca, A. Macciocchi, M. Aapro10.1093/annonc/mdg417Annals of Oncology

[33] Comparative activity of anti-emetic drugs 2007Karin Jordan, Hans J. Schmoll, Matti S. Aapro10.1016/j.critrevonc.2006.08.003Critical Reviews in Oncology/Hematology

[34] Anti-emetic activity of corticosteroids in patients receiving cancer chemotherapy: dosing, efficacy, and tolerability analysis 2007S.M. Grunberg10.1093/annonc/mdl347Annals of Oncology

[35] Efficacy and Tolerability of Aprepitant for the Prevention of Chemotherapy-Induced Nausea and Vomiting in Patients With Breast Cancer After Moderately Emetogenic Chemotherapy 2005David G. Warr, Paul J. Hesketh, Richard J. Gralla, Hyman B. Muss, Jørn Herrstedt, Peter D. Eisenberg, Harry Raftopoulos, Steven M. Grunberg, Munir Gabriel, Anthony Rodgers, Norman Bohidar, George Klinger, Carolyn M. Hustad, Kevin J. Horgan, Franck Skobieranda10.1200/jco.2005.09.050Journal of Clinical Oncology

[36] Randomized, Double-Blind, Dose- Finding Study of Dexamethasone in Preventing Acute Emesis Induced by Anthracyclines, Carboplatin, or Cyclophosphamide: 200410.1200/jco.2004.09.040Journal of Clinical Oncology

[37] Double-blind, dose-finding study of four intravenous doses of dexamethasone in the prevention of cisplatin-induced acute emesis. Italian Group for Anti-emetic Research. 199810.1200/jco.1998.16.9.2937Journal of Clinical Oncology

[38] The Oral Neurokinin-1 Antagonist Aprepitant for the Prevention of Chemotherapy-Induced Nausea and Vomiting: A Multinational, Randomized, Double-Blind, Placebo-Controlled Trial in Patients Receiving High-Dose Cisplatin—The Aprepitant Protocol 052 Study Group 2003Paul J. Hesketh, Steven M.

Grunberg, Richard J. Gralla, David G. Warr, Fausto Roila, Ronald de Wit, Sant P. Chawla, Alexandra D. Carides, Juliana Ianus, Mary E. Elmer, Judith K. Evans, Klaus Beck, Scott Reines, Kevin J. Horgan10.1200/jco.2003.01.095Journal of Clinical Oncology

[39] Addition of the neurokinin 1 receptor antagonist aprepitant to standard anti-emetic therapy improves control of chemotherapy-induced nausea and vomiting 2003Sergio Poli-Bigelli, Jose Rodrigues-Pereira, Alexandra D. Carides, Guoguang Julie Ma, Krista Eldridge, Anita Hipple, Judith K. Evans, Kevin J. Horgan, Francesca Lawson, 10.1002/cncr.11433Cancer

[40] Comparison of an aprepitant regimen with a multiple-day ondansetron regimen, both with dexamethasone, for anti- emetic efficacy in high-dose cisplatin treatment 2006H.J. Schmoll, M.S. Aapro, S. Poli-Bigelli, H.-K. Kim, K. Park, K. Jordan, J. von Pawel, H. Giezek, T. Ahmed, C.Y. Chan10.1093/annonc/mdl019Annals of Oncology

[41] Lack of effect of aprepitant on the pharmacokinetics of docetaxel in cancer patients 2005Peter Nygren, Kenneth Hande, Kevin J. Petty, Margaret Fedgchin, Kristien van Dyck, Anup Majumdar, Debbie Panebianco, Marina de Smet, Tuli Ahmed, M. Gail Murphy, Keith M. Gottesdiener, Veronique Cocquyt, Simon van Belle10.1007/s00280-004-0946-3Cancer Chemotherapy and Pharmacology

[42] Comparison of three protracted anti- emetic regimens for the control of delayed emesis in cisplatin-treated patients 1992Isabel Moreno, Rafael Rosell, Albert Abad, Agusti Barnadas, Joan Carles, Nuria Ribelles, Victoria Solano, Albert Font10.1016/0959-8049(92)90515- 4European Journal of Cancer

[43] Controlling delayed vomiting: double- blind, randomized trial comparing placebo, dexamethasone alone, and metoclopramide plus dexamethasone in patients receiving cisplatin. 1989M G Kris, R J Gralla, L B Tyson, R A Clark, C Cirrincione, S Groshen10.1200/jco.1989.7.1.108Journal of Clinical Oncology

[44] A comparative analysis of the potential of cannabinoids and ondansetron to suppress cisplatin-induced emesis in the *Suncus murinus* (house musk shrew) 2004Magdalena Kwiatkowska, LindaA. Parker, Page Burton, Raphael Mechoulam10.1007/s00213-003-1739-9Psychopharmacology

[45] Regulation of nausea and vomiting by cannabinoids, 2011Linda A Parker, Erin M Rock, Cheryl L Limebeer10.1111/j.1476-5381.2010.01176.xBritish Journal of Pharmacology

[46] Update on anti-emetics for chemotherapy-induced emesis 2005I. N. Olver10.1111/j.1445-5004.2005.00879.xInternal Medicine Journal

[47] anti-emetic placebo: Reduce adverse drug interactions between chemotherapeutic agents and anti-emetic drugs in cancer patients, 2008Zhongyi Zhang, Yong Wang, Yan Wang, Feng, Xu10.1016/j.mehy.2007.06.029Medical Hypotheses

[48] Premedication with H1 and H2 blocking agents reduces the incidence of postoperative nausea and vomiting 2004A.W. Doenicke, R. Hoernecke, I. Celik10.1007/s00011-004-0367-0Inflammation Research

[49] Radioreceptor Binding Profile of the Atypical Antipsychotic Olanzapine 1996Frank P Bymaster, David O Calligaro, Julie F Falcone, Richard D Marsh, Nicholas A Moore, Nicholas C Tye, Philip Seeman, David T Wong10.1016/0893-133x(94)00129-nNeuropsychopharmacology

[50] A phase II trial of olanzapine for the prevention of chemotherapy-induced

nausea and vomiting: A Hoosier Oncology Group study 2005Rudolph M. Navari, Lawrence H. Einhorn, Steven D. Passik, Patrick J. Loehrer, Cynthia Johnson, M. L. Mayer, J. McClean, Jake Vinson, W. Pletcher10.1007/s00520-004-0755-6Supportive Care in Cancer

[51] A phase II trial of olanzapine, dexamethasone, and palonosetron for the prevention of chemotherapy-induced nausea and vomiting: a Hoosier oncology group study 2007Rudolph M. Navari, Lawrence H. Einhorn, Patrick J. Loehrer, Steven D. Passik, Jake Vinson, John McClean, Naveed Chowhan, Nasser H. Hanna, Cynthia S. Johnson10.1007/s00520-007-0248-5Supportive Care in Cancer.

[52] Treatment of Breakthrough and Refractory Chemotherapy-Induced Nausea and Vomiting 2015Rudolph M. Navari10.1155/2015/595894BioMed Research International

[53] Anti-emetics: American Society of Clinical Oncology Clinical Practice Guideline Update Summary 2017Paul J. Hesketh, Kari Bohlke, Mark G. Kris10.1200/jop.2017.026351Journal of Oncology Practice

[54] Medication Error Factors, Safety Guideline System, Flow of Drug Usage, and Code of Conduct to Prevent Medication Error, 2018, Arvidareyna Panca, Nikma Fitriasari, Wiwik Supartiwi 10.11594/bbrj.01.02.01, Bioinformatics and Biomedical Research Journal

Chapter 6

Small Molecule/HLA Complexes Alter the Cellular Proteomic Content

Gia-Gia Toni Hò, Wiebke Hiemisch, Andreas Pich, Michelle Matern, Lareen Sophi Gräser, Rainer Blasczyk, Christina Bade-Doeding and Gwendolin Sabrina Simper

Abstract

A medical product usually undergoes several clinical trials, including the testing of volunteers. Nevertheless, genomic variances in the patients cannot be considered comprehensively and adverse drug reactions (ADRs) are missed or misinterpreted during trials. Despite the relation between ADRs and human leukocyte antigen (HLA) molecules being known for several years, the fundamental molecular mechanisms leading to the development of such an ADR often remains only vaguely solved. The analysis of the peptidome can reveal changes in peptide presentation post-drug treatment and explain, for example, the severe cutaneous ADR in HLA-B*57:01-positive patients treated with the antiretroviral drug abacavir in anti-HIV therapy. However, as seen in the biophysical features of HLA-A*31:01-presented peptides, treatment with the anticonvulsant carbamazepine only induces minor changes. Since the binding of a drug to a certain HLA allelic variant is extremely distinct, the influence of the small molecule/protein complex on the proteomic content of a cell becomes clear. A sophisticated methodology elucidating the impact of drug treatment on cells is a full proteome analysis. The principal component analysis of abacavir, carbamazepine or carbamazepine-10,11-epoxid treated cells reveals clear clustering of the drug-treated and the untreated samples that express the respective HLA molecule. Following drug treatment, several proteins were shown to be significantly up- or downregulated. Proteomics and peptidomics are valuable tools to differential clinical outcomes of patients with the same HLA phenotype.

Keywords: Adverse drug reaction, human leukocyte antigen, abacavir, carbamazepine, proteome

1. Introduction

Since treatment with drugs can trigger harmful adverse events, several tests have to be performed before the approval of new drugs. In preclinical trials, the substance is tested in cell culture or animal experiments in order to ascertain its pharmacokinetics, the pharmacodynamics and to exclude any toxic effects. Clinical trials are designed for the examination of the efficacy and safety of a drug under defined parameters; they are differentiated into different stages [1]. Clinical trials can be randomized, masked, placebo-controlled or crossover studies. Therefore, they are favored towards non-interventional case–control studies [2].

Phase 0 studies are first-in-human-studies using subtherapeutic dosage of the tested drug in a small group of fewer than 15 healthy volunteers to asses pharmacokinetics and pharmacodynamics [3]. In phase I studies therapeutic dosages of the drug are tested in healthy volunteers to examine its tolerability and safety [4]. They are not randomized trials, making them susceptible for selection bias [5]. Phase II studies are more broadly conceived, and the drug is tested in sick individuals for spotting its efficacy, optimal doses and tolerability, including potential side effects. This same occurs in phase III studies where several thousands of volunteers are tested in order to prove a significant therapeutic effect of the drug under study. After drug's approval, the pharmacovigilance can still be monitored in the so-called post-marketing surveillance trials or phase IV studies [3].

Despite these different stages of testing, genomic variances in the patients cannot be considered completely. While differences in metabolism are easier to spot, there are other genes not being taken into account, thus leading to the lack of some adverse drug reactions (ADRs) in clinical trials [6].

2. Adverse drug reactions (ADRs)

2.1 ADRs as an underestimated factor in the health care system

If harm is occurring during treatment with a drug, it can be termed as an adverse event (AE), regardless of a causal link between the drug usage and the symptoms. However, adverse drug events (ADEs) are caused by the drug application [7–9]. This includes harm triggered by the substance itself, as well as harm induced by inappropriate dosages or premature discontinuation of the medication [7, 10]. For example, the overdose of a drug is an ADE. Depending on the drug, the probability of occurring an ADE differs, being very low in patients treated with for instance with antimitotics, and very high in patients under immunosuppressive medication [11]. This is explicable by the mode of action of the drug, for instance the antimitotic nystatin attaches to the cell membrane of fungal cells causing their disruption, but does not disrupt human cells. Contrarily, immunosuppressive medication may led a patients to be more prone to infections and cancer, since the whole immune system is suppressed [10].

Despite a correct dosage and application, unintended and harmful reactions to drugs can still occur [12]. Such ADRs are distinguished from side effects that comprise positive, negative and irrelevant unintended effects [7, 10, 11].

ADRs can be classified into dose-dependent and predictable type A and dose-independent idiosyncratic type B [13] (see **Figure 1**). Most ADRs are type A reactions (>80%), explicable by the pharmacological activity of the drug [13, 14]. Therefore, they can occur in nearly all patients [14]. Type A ADRs are rarely fatal, and the symptoms are drug-specific [13–15]. These ADRs are affected by drug pharmacokinetics, comorbidities and drug–drug-interactions [14]. In contrast to type B ADRs, the emergence of type A ADRs are comprehensible [10]. At the first appearance, type B ADRs seem to be idiosyncratic, but the immune system is often involved and, in these cases, they are called drug hypersensitivity reactions [10]. The clinical picture can involve a single organ or be systemic [16]. Despite their less frequent occurrence, type B ADRs are characterized by an increased mortality rate [13, 14].

Type B ADRs can be subclassified depending on the drug's mode of action with immune cells into allergic, pharmacologic and pseudoallergic reactions [14].

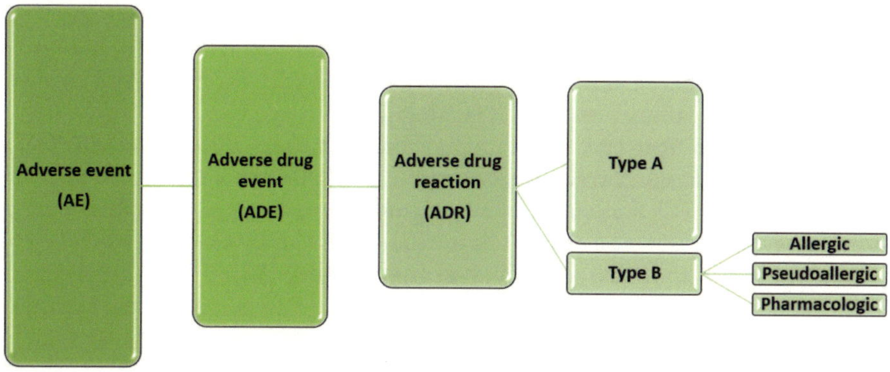

Figure 1.
Classification of ADRs. ADRs are ADEs that occur despite a proper dosage and application, and are mainly subclassified into type A and rare type B reactions.

Hereby, allergic reactions are mediated by both the innate, as well as by the adaptive immune systems and include, for instance, the IgE-mediated penicillin allergy or contact dermatitis. Pseudoallergic reactions manifest, for example, as urticaria/anaphylaxis bronchospasm. Pharmacologic reactions are T cell-mediated. Other possible classifications are relative to the time point of the first symptoms, or to their type of immune mechanism or type of drug [14].

The ADRs have often arisen as an underestimated factor in the health care system, due to their underreporting and underdiagnosis [15, 17–20].

2.2 Type B ADRs manifest as different clinical pictures

Type B ADRs can be systemic or affect certain organs, with skin, liver and blood cells being the most impacted [16]. Cutaneous forms of ADRs include, for example, maculopapular exanthema (MPE), acute generalized exanthematous pustulosis (AGEP), drug reaction with eosinophilia and systemic symptoms (DRESS), Stevens-Johnson syndrome (SJS) and toxic epidermal necrolysis (TEN) [10].

The MPE is relatively mild, forming rashes with macules or erythematous and maculopapular lesions [21, 22].

AGEP is known to have an acute onset characterized by fever, large erythema and sterile, non-follicular pinhead-sized rapidly appearing pustules with desquamation starting from four to ten days later [10, 23]. The mucosa is barely involved; other organs are free of symptoms. Several drugs are shown to induce AGEP, among which we can find aminopenicillins, quinolones and pristinamycine [10, 23].

The DRESS, also known as drug-induced delayed multiple organ hypersensitivity syndrome (DIDMOHS), drug-induced hypersensitivity syndrome (DIHS), drug hypersensitivity syndrome (DHS) or hypersensitivity syndrome (HSS), is characterized by a cutaneous exanthema spread for over more than half of the body and other organ's involvement, such as hepatitis, eosinophilia, arthralgia or lymphadenopathy [10, 24]. DRESS can be triggered by anticonvulsants (carbamazepine (CBZ), oxcarbazepine, lamotrigine, phenytoin and phenobarbital), sulfonamides and uricostatic drugs (allopurinol) [24].

Although overall SJS and TEN may be fatal in 20–25% of all cases, in TEN the mortality may increase up to 48% and, in the elderly, TEN can be fatal in 70% [24, 25]. Typically, SJS/TEN manifest with skin blisters and bullae, detachment of the skin and erosions of mucous membranes [26]. In SJS, up to 10% of the body surface area is affected, while in TEN at least 30% is affected; if between 10% and 30% of the body surface area are affected a transitional form is diagnosed [25].

Additionally, complications with the lungs, fever and hypovolemia may occur [25]. It has been shown that apoptotic signal-associated cytokine levels are increased in SJS/TEN [27]. Patients suffering from SJS/TEN are positive for Nikolsky's sign, yet specific laboratory parameters are still lacking [28].

The algorithm of drug causality for epidermal necrolysis algorithm (ALDEN) is designed to ascertain the correct diagnosis [29]. SJS/TEN can be triggered not only by anticonvulsive medication (CBZ, lamotrigine, phenytoin and phenobarbital), sulfonamides and uricostatic drugs (allopurinol), but also by oxicam-NSAIDs, sulfasalazine and antiretroviral medication (nevirapine) [30].

3. Associations of human leukocyte antigen (HLA) alleles with type B ADRs

Associations of certain alleles of the human leukocyte antigen (HLA) system with type B ADRs have been previously reported [31]. The HLA molecules are cell surface glycoproteins that present peptides to immune cells exerting their crucial function in the recognition of self/non-self. By varying in their function and structure, HLA class I and II molecules can be differentiated. Whereas HLA class II molecules are composed of two membrane-anchored chains α and β, HLA class I molecules are composed of the invariant light chain β_2-microglobulin (β_2m) non-covalently linked to the membrane-anchored heavy α-chain [32]. The peptide-binding groove of the HLA class I molecules is formed by the α1 and α2 domains, where a peptide with a length of eight to ten amino acids is presented. Contrarily, HLA class II molecules present longer peptides, since their peptide-binding groove formed by the α1 and the ß1 domains is open in both ends. HLA class I molecules interact with $CD8^+$ T cells and present peptides of intracellular origin, whereby HLA class II molecules display peptides derived from the extracellular space or from vesicles to interact with $CD4^+$ T cells [33]. As part of the adaptive immune system, T cells are able to scan cells for the presence of antigens inducing the death of the respective cells, or releasing of cytokines leading to the activation of other immune cells. Some differences can also be found in the expression patterns of HLA molecules. While HLA class I is expressed by all nucleated cells and platelets, HLA class II expression is limited to immune cells, such as antigen presenting cells, macrophages and B cells [32, 34].

The HLA molecules are characterized by an exceptional polygenism and polymorphism [35]. The HLA genes are encoded in a 220-genes-encompassing region organized in HLA class I, class II and class III genes, whereby class III genes are immune system-related [32, 35, 36]. Among the currently known 28,786 alleles, 20,597 are HLA class I alleles and 7,723 are HLA class II alleles, making it impossible to consider allelic variants in clinical trials [35]. Therefore, HLA-mediated ADRs are inevitably overlooked before the approval of the drug.

As such, the association of abacavir (ABC) hypersensitivity with HLA-B*57:01 is the best known [37]. About 5% of HIV patients that are treated with ABC show symptoms [38, 39]. Other examples are the association of CBZ hypersensitivity with two alleles, HLA-A*31:01 and HLA-B*15:02, and of allopurinol hypersensitivity with HLA-B*58:01 [22, 40, 41]. In Han Chinese, all patients developing CBZ hypersensitivity were positive for HLA-B*15:02 [41]. In Northern Europeans, in the presence of the allele HLA-A*31:01, the risk for an ADR increases from 5–26%, whereas in its absence it decreases to 3.8% [22]. Moreover, the association of ticlopidine, nevirapine and/or dapsone hypersensitivity with the alleles HLA-A*33:03, HLA-DRB1*01:01 and HLA-B*13:01 has also been described [42–44] (see **Figure 2**). In general, ADRs can occur in about 15% of the patients during hospitalization [52].

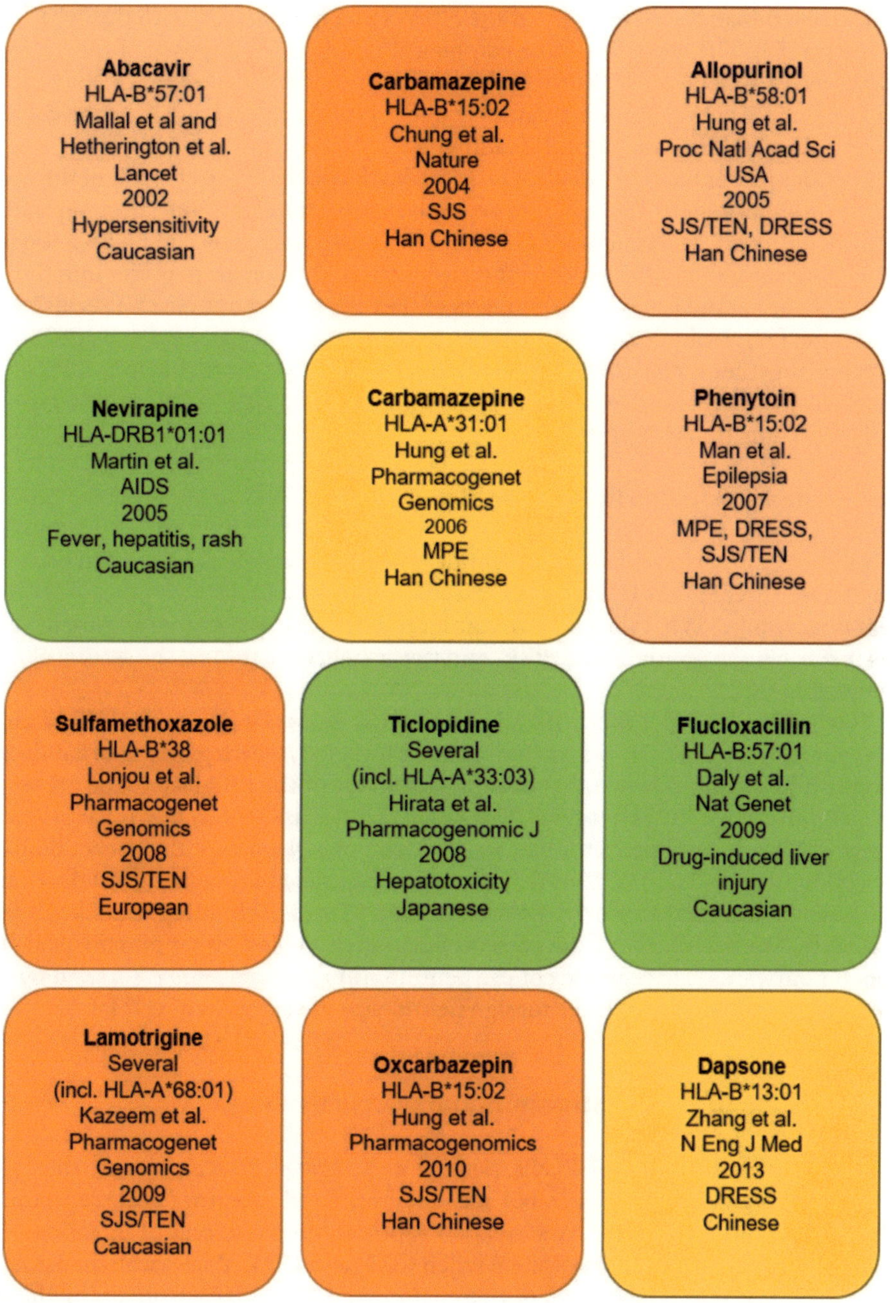
Abacavir
HLA-B*57:01
Mallal et al and
Hetherington et al.
Lancet
2002
Hypersensitivity
Caucasian
Carbamazepine
HLA-B*15:02
Chung et al.
Nature
2004
SJS
Han Chinese
Allopurinol
HLA-B*58:01
Hung et al.
Proc Natl Acad Sci
USA
2005
SJS/TEN, DRESS
Han Chinese
Nevirapine
HLA-DRB1*01:01
Martin et al.
AIDS
2005
Fever, hepatitis, rash
Caucasian
Carbamazepine
HLA-A*31:01
Hung et al.
Pharmacogenet
Genomics
2006
MPE
Han Chinese
Phenytoin
HLA-B*15:02
Man et al.
Epilepsia
2007
MPE, DRESS,
SJS/TEN
Han Chinese
Sulfamethoxazole
HLA-B*38
Lonjou et al.
Pharmacogenet
Genomics
2008
SJS/TEN
European
Ticlopidine
Several
(incl. HLA-A*33:03)
Hirata et al.
Pharmacogenomic J
2008
Hepatotoxicity
Japanese
Flucloxacillin
HLA-B:57:01
Daly et al.
Nat Genet
2009
Drug-induced liver
injury
Caucasian
Lamotrigine
Several
(incl. HLA-A*68:01)
Kazeem et al.
Pharmacogenet
Genomics
2009
SJS/TEN
Caucasian
Oxcarbazepin
HLA-B*15:02
Hung et al.
Pharmacogenomics
2010
SJS/TEN
Han Chinese
Dapsone
HLA-B*13:01
Zhang et al.
N Eng J Med
2013
DRESS
Chinese

Figure 2.
Depiction of some HLA-associated ADRs. Each example box includes the name of the drug, the associated HLA allele, the author of the first publication, the journal and year of the publication, the syndromes and adverse reactions (SJS/TEN in orange, MPE and DRESS in yellow, hepatotoxicity/drug-induced liver toxicity in green, mixed symptoms in light orange) and the population where the association was observed. Among others the following drugs were shown to be associated with ADRs: Abacavir [37, 45], carbamazepine [41, 46], allopurinol [40], nevirapine [44], phenytoin [47], sulfamethoxazole [48], ticlopidine [42], flucloxacillin [49], lamotrigine [50], oxcarbazepine [51], dapsone [43].

3.1 Peptide loading of HLA class I molecules

Peptide loading occurs in the endoplasmic reticulum after biosynthesis and folding of the nascent HLA class I heavy chain. The interaction with the chaperone calnexin stabilizes the association of the HLA class I heavy chain with the light chain β_2m [53]. The peptide loading complex (PLC) is also composed of the chaperone calreticulin, the transmembrane glycoprotein tapasin and the thiol oxidoreductase endoplasmic reticulum resident protein 57, which ensure the correct glycosylation, folding and peptide loading [54].

Peptides presented by HLA class I molecules derive from the cytosol. In the cytosol, ubiquitinylated proteins are degraded via proteasomes into short peptides with a length of 3–22 amino acids [32, 55]. The transporter associated with antigen processing subserves ATP-dependent translocation of cytosolic peptides into the lumen of the endoplasmic reticulum, where they are loaded onto the HLA class I molecule [32]. Ubiquitinylated proteins are composed of misfolded and aged proteins, together with defective ribosomal products, that comprise up to 30% of the newly synthesized proteins [56, 57]. Thereby, a rapid CD8$^+$ T cell reaction is enabled in infections [58].

3.2 Peptide presentation by HLA class I molecules

As already described above, the peptide binding region (PBR) is shaped by the α1 and α2 regions of HLA class I molecules, and the α1 and ß1 regions of HLA class II molecules. What they have in common is the basic structure composed of a β-sheet at the ground of the PBR, and two α-helices that form the sidewise boundaries [32].

Solely those peptides with a certain amino acid sequence fit into the PBR of an HLA allele. HLA alleles mostly differ in the PBR region, which gives them a unique peptide binding motif, since alterations in the shape of the PBR lead to the presentation of an altered set of peptides. The PBR of HLA class I molecules is partitioned into pockets A-F, with pocket A binding residue 1 of a given peptide, pocket B binding residue 2 and so on [36, 59–61]. Typically, a peptide binding motif is defined by a N- and a C-terminal anchor, the amino acids at p2 and pΩ binding to pocket B and F [32, 61]. The side chains of the presented peptide can bind either into the pockets or point outwards. This complex of the peptide and HLA molecule is scanned by T cells that are able to recognize foreign peptides in the complex of self HLA.

4. Activation of the adaptive immune system by drugs

During the maturation of T cells, positive and negative selection assure the generation of an HLA-restricted, but self-tolerant, T cell receptor (TCR) repertoire. Therefore, viral, bacterial or stress-related peptides present in case of infection are recognized by the immune system when CD8$^+$ and CD4$^+$ T cells scan the HLA molecules. The TCR is composed of two chains, α and β, with each obtaining three complementarity determining regions (CDRs) named CDR1, CDR2 and CDR3. These are extremely variable loops able to recognize both the combination of the HLA molecule and the peptide [32].

For the activation of CD8$^+$ T cells, not only the interaction of the TCR is necessary, but also the interaction of the CD8 co-receptor with the HLA molecule, leading to the phosphorylation of the immunoreceptor tyrosine-based activation motifs [62, 63]. As a second signal, the CD28 molecules on naïve T cells need to interact with a receptor of the B7 family on the target cell, aiming to ensure their survival. Finally, cytokines initiate the third signal by triggering the clonal expansion and differentiation into effector cells. The activated cytotoxic T cell can cause the apoptosis of the target cell through the release of granules with perforin, granzymes, and a scaffold protein triggering the activation of the caspase 3 [64].

Synthetical drugs usually only have a size of less than one kDa, making them invisible to the immune system. Nevertheless, they can induce a reaction within the immune system through their binding to a carrier protein (hapten), or after metabolization of the drug (prohapten) [21]. This hapten-protein complex can trigger several immune reactions, from type I to IV, according to Gell and Coombs [14]. The binding of IgE antibodies to the complex activates mastcells and basophils in type I reactions [14, 21]. This can be seen, for example, in allergy caused by β-lactam antibiotics manifesting as urticarial and anaphylaxis [14]. Type II reactions are mediated by IgG and IgM antibody-dependent cell-mediated cytotoxicity, and are seen in aminopyrine hypersensitivity leading to leukopenia. On the other hand, type III reactions are characterized by IgG-driven immune-complexes that are deposited or cleared by complement activation [10, 14, 21]. A type III reaction example is the minocycline-mediated DRESS [10]. Delayed type IV reactions are generally triggered by T cells.

T cells have been isolated from the blister fluid of patients suffering from cutaneous ADRs [65, 66]. Three models (1, 2 and 3) tend to explain the involvement of cytotoxic T cells in HLA class I-associated ADRs.

1. In the first model, called the hapten/prohapten model, the drug or its metabolite can bind as hapten either to a peptide that is later presented in the context of self-HLA, or to a protein that is processed and subsequently presented as a modified self-peptide [67–71]. This has been shown in cases of allergy to β-lactam antibiotics that are B and T cell-mediated; the hapten binds to lysine side chains of presented peptides [72–75]. Moreover, T cell proliferation and toxicity are induced by a reactive nitroso metabolite of the antibiotic sulfamethoxazole, which is able to bind to peptides that are presented in the context of self-HLA [76].

2. The second model is the pharmacological-interaction (p-i) model that initiates the fast and direct activation of cytotoxic T cells, independently from the metabolism and peptide processing, by a noncovalent interaction of the drug with the HLA molecule and/or the TCR. The reversible and potentially weak interaction established between the drug and the immune receptors induces functional changes in the conformation of the immune receptors [77, 78]. In the case of allergies caused by sulfamethoxazole, the p-I models can also be applied, since T cells can be stimulated with fixed sulfamethoxazole-treated cells, being possible to wash the drug off afterwards [79, 80].

3. In the third model, the altered repertoire model, the binding of the drug to the PBR of the HLA molecule induces an alteration in its shape and ability to present peptides, so that an altered peptide repertoire is selected and recognized as foreign [81, 82]. This is seen in ABC hypersensitivity, where the drug binds to the F pocket of HLA-B*57:01, thus triggering an alteration in the pΩ anchor [83, 84].

5. Analysis of the peptidome in HLA-associated ADRs

The drug ABC is a guanosine-analogue indicated for HIV therapy. ABC hypersensitivity manifests as a systemic disease, striking up 11 days upon start of the treatment [37]. Fever, rash, constitutional symptoms, and gastrointestinal symptoms, such as nausea, vomiting, diarrhea, or abdominal pain, characterize the clinical picture of ABC hypersensitivity [37, 39]. In 2002, its association with

HLA-B*57:01 has been published [37, 45] and in 2008, the testing for the presence of HLA-B*57:01 in patients was recommended to reduce the risk of ABC hypersensitivity [39].

In order to prove or disprove the altered repertoire model, analysis of the peptidome has been performed. Furthermore, it is also possible to unravel the structure of the drug bound to the HLA molecule, by using a peptide found in the analysis of the peptidome. In ABC hypersensitivity, both experiments were performed. The crystal structure of ABC bound to the F pocket of HLA-B*57:01 has shown that this position is already occupied by the drug, thus leading to an alteration in the peptidome [83]. Typically, peptides presented by HLA-B*57:01 are anchored by a C-terminal tryptophan, tyrosine or phenylalanine [83, 84]. The alteration in the chemical properties of the PBR enables binding of a new repertoire of endogenous self-peptides [83, 84]. These peptides will then trigger the activation of ABC-specific cytotoxic T cells, resulting in ABC hypersensitivity [83].

The drug CBZ is a tricyclic anticonvulsant usually used in the therapy of bipolar disorders, as well as in nerve pain [21, 85–88]. Certain patients treated with CBZ can develop severe SJS/TEN, DRESS or MPE, as recognized soon after the approval of the drug [86, 89]. Later on, the association of CBZ-mediated SJS/TEN with HLA-B*15:02 became evident, primarily in South East Asian populations [41, 90–92]. Interestingly, in Caucasians and some Asian populations, milder symptoms, such as DRESS and MPE, were found to be associated with HLA-A*31:01 [22, 81, 93, 94]. As the allele HLA-B*15:02 is mostly found in South Asia, being nearly absent in Europe [95], this may explain why the HLA-B*15:02 is not found in Caucasians with CBZ hypersensitivity [96]. Contrarily, the allele HLA-A*31:01 has been shown to be distributed worldwide [95]. Despite clearly differing in their sequence in the PBR, both alleles are associated with CBZ hypersensitivity [21]. However, research has shown that CBZ hypersensitivity is presented as two distinct diseases forms with differing mechanisms of action [21], consistent with the different clinical pictures and median onset of HLA-B*15:02- and HLA-A*31:01-associated CBZ hypersensitivity [24, 95].

The altered repertoire model has been discussed for the association of HLA-B*15:02 with CBZ-mediated SJS/TEN, but no clear alterations in the peptidome, after treatment with CBZ, were found [83, 97, 98]. Additionally, derivates of CBZ have been shown to bind soluble immobilized HLA-B*15:02 [99]. Later published studies have revealed that the main metabolite CBZ-10,11-epoxide (EPX) was binding to the F pocket, so that the nonpolar aromatic pΩ anchor was no longer able to bind that position [81]. These findings are in agreement with those where a polymorphism in the epoxide hydroxylase 1 was influencing the risk of SJS/TEN in the Han Chinese population [100]. Nevertheless, this does not explain the activation of CBZ-specific T cells *in vitro* [99, 101].

In HLA-A*31:01-associated CBZ-mediated ADRs, no clear alterations in the peptide binding motif post CBZ and EPX treatment have been found [21].

6. Analysis of the proteome in HLA-associated ADRs

The field of proteomics greatly contributes to a comprehensive profiling of the immune response. To enable side effect predictions for uncharacterized drugs, and to prevent the delay in the licensing process, one widely used action is the analysis of drug (small molecule)-protein interactions [102].

Small molecules-targeted proteins [103] are clearly disturbed or even enabled on their protein–protein-interaction networks. The ability of a protein to initiate the onset of expression, regulation, and/or function of its cognate interaction partner, highly depends on its structural integrity. Drugs are not only physically, but also functionally, involved with many other proteins and cellular components, as both drugs and proteins are embedded in cellular pathways and networks [103]. The identification of regulated proteins following drug treatment provides insight into the regulatory impact of drugs on target cells (see **Figure 3**). The classical HLA-Ia molecules, one of the molecular interaction partners of small molecules, are genetically very polymorphic and structurally highly variable. This variability is attributed to the peptide repertoire that can be intracellularly selected and extracellularly presented by the distinct HLA-Ia molecules. This structural variability

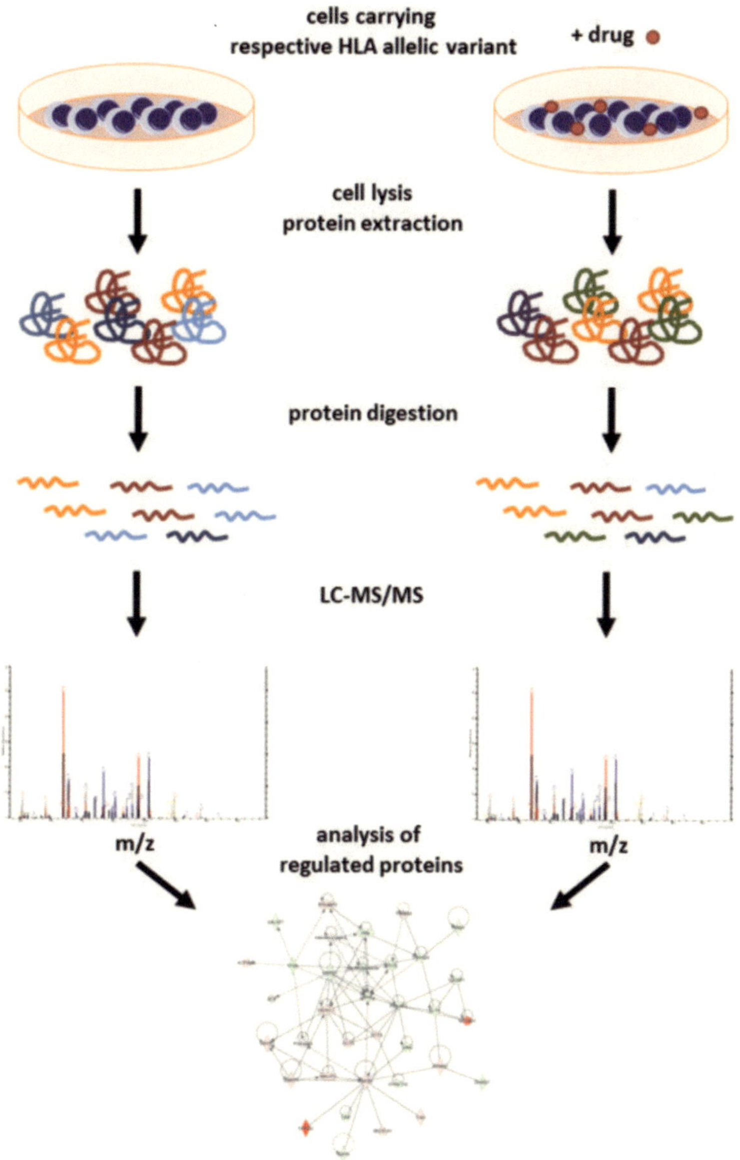

Figure 3.
Workflow of protein drug profiling. Comprehensive analysis of protein abundance in drug-treated cells compared to control cells. After drug treatment, the cells were lysed, and proteins extracted from the sample. Proteins were digested into peptides and analyzed by liquid chromatography coupled to tandem mass spectrometry (LC–MS/MS). Significant regulated proteins were determined and analyzed via pathway analysis.

makes molecular and bioinformatical analyses of drug-HLA interaction calculations impossible. Unfortunately, the binding of a drug to an HLA-Ia molecule has a profound impact on certain HLA-allele carriers [97]. To somehow enable bioinformatic calculations, experimental achievements in the analysis of small molecule-protein interactions showed broad alterations in the proteome repertoire of targeted cells [21]. Proteomic analysis provides information on protein expression, and mass spectrometry (MS)-based protein drug profiling, improves the understanding of presentable peptides and identification of HLA-bound ligands [104].

ABC-mediated ADRs in HLA-B*57:01 positive individuals are unique in their rapid emergence [105]. Although it could be possible to demonstrate that ABC alters the chemical properties of the PBR, and elicits immune responses through ABC-specific T cells, not all HLA-B*57:01 positive individuals develop ABC-induced hypersensitivity reactions [39]. It becomes obvious that not only the HLA type, but also further individual patient-specific factors, may contribute to ABC-mediated ADRs. The proteome analysis of ABC-treated cells provides insights into the regulatory impact of ABC in the HLA-B*57:01-expressing cells (see **Figure 4**). ABC treatment resulted in an increased apoptosis rate; proteins that generally lead to decreased viral replication were differentially regulated, such as PML and TNPO3. Furthermore, ABC treatment provided hints towards an increased proteasomal degradation activity that would enlarge the pool of presentable peptides. The proteomic drug profiling of ABC-treated cells allowed to enlarge the knowledge about ABC-dependent cellular changes.

CBZ-mediated ADRs are associated with HLA-A*31:01 and HLA-B*15:02. A recent study about HLA-B*15:02-restricted CBZ-induced ADRs revealed that EPX, as the main metabolite, might be responsible for severe reactions in HLA-B*15:02-positive individuals [81, 99]. To increase the understanding of differential clinical courses, proteome analysis of CBZ- and EPX-treated cells has been performed [21]. CBZ treatment of HLA-A*31:01-positive cells provided evidence towards an increased ubiquitination activity, but with a stable cellular viability. On the other hand, EPX treatment of HLA-B*15:02-positive cells resulted in increased cytokine

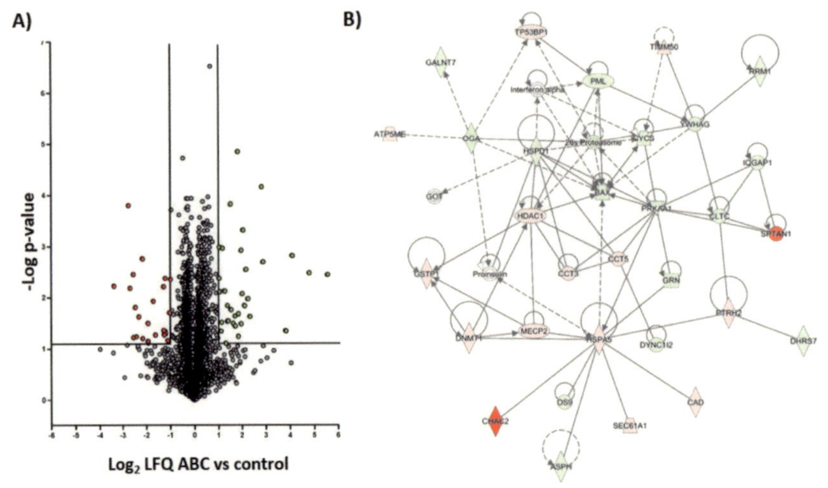

Figure 4.
Mass spectrometric analysis of the proteome of Abacavir (ABC) treated and non-treated cells. A) Protein abundance after ABC treatment. Significantly upregulated proteins are shown in green and downregulated proteins are shown in red. B) Network analysis for up- and downregulated protein groups following ABC treatment. Upregulated proteins are illustrated in red, downregulated proteins are illustrated in green; non-colored proteins were added by the IPA algorithm. High confident interactions are represented by a continuous line; medium confident interactions are represented by a dashed line.

release [21]. The proteomic analyses of CBZ and EPX-treated cells provided the first perceptions into the potential protein regulation and involvement of cellular pathways. Furthermore, proteomic profiling has also shown to contribute to the comprehensive understanding of CBZ-induced ADRs in the context of HLA specificity.

A deep knowledge over the spectrum of proteins that are influenced by drug/protein complexes clearly plays an important role in drug safety, and offers the possibility to identify potential toxicity targets. The emerging role of proteomics improves personalization of immunotherapy treatment in HLA- associated diseases, since detail target analysis supports the understanding of enigmatic HLA-associated ADRs.

7. Conclusions

The proteomic repertoire is a real time view on the health status of a cell, and can be altered through the medical condition of the illness after treatment with the respective drug. Therefore, the knowledge of the proteomic repertoire of a healthy cell pre- and post-treatment with a given drug is indispensable and should not be underestimated.

Acknowledgements

We would like to thank Karsten Heidrich and Ulrike Schrameck for their excellent technical assistance in the mass spectrometry analysis.

Conflict of interest

The authors declare no conflict of interest.

Author details

Gia-Gia Toni Hò[1], Wiebke Hiemisch[1], Andreas Pich[2], Michelle Matern[1], Lareen Sophi Gräser[1], Rainer Blasczyk[1], Christina Bade-Doeding[1] and Gwendolin Sabrina Simper[1*]

1 Institute for Transfusion Medicine and Transplant Engineering, Medical School Hannover, Hannover, Germany

2 Institute for Toxicology, Medical School Hannover, Hannover, Germany

*Address all correspondence to: simper.gwendolin@mh-hannover.de

References

[1] Ramalhinho AC, Castelo-Branco M. Preparation of an Academic Clinical Trial. Methods in molecular biology. 2021;2197:317-330.

[2] Umscheid CA, Margolis DJ, Grossman CE. Key concepts of clinical trials: a narrative review. Postgraduate medicine. 2011;123(5):194-204.

[3] Phase 0 trials: a platform for drug development? Lancet. 2009;374(9685):176.

[4] Le Tourneau C, Lee JJ, Siu LL. Dose escalation methods in phase I cancer clinical trials. Journal of the National Cancer Institute. 2009;101(10):708-720.

[5] Eynde BJVd, Baren Nv, Baurain J-F. Is There a Clinical Future for IDO1 Inhibitors After the Failure of Epacadostat in Melanoma? Annual Review of Cancer Biology. 2020;4(1):241-256.

[6] Naranjo CA, Busto U, Sellers EM. Difficulties in assessing adverse drug reactions in clinical trials. Progress in neuro-psychopharmacology & biological psychiatry. 1982;6(4-6):651-657.

[7] Nebeker JR, Barach P, Samore MH. Clarifying adverse drug events: a clinician's guide to terminology, documentation, and reporting. Annals of internal medicine. 2004;140(10):795-801.

[8] Gurwitz JH, Field TS, Avorn J, McCormick D, Jain S, Eckler M, et al. Incidence and preventability of adverse drug events in nursing homes. The American journal of medicine. 2000;109(2):87-94.

[9] Bates DW, Cullen DJ, Laird N, Petersen LA, Small SD, Servi D, et al. Incidence of adverse drug events and potential adverse drug events. Implications for prevention. ADE Prevention Study Group. Jama. 1995;274(1):29-34.

[10] Simper G, Celik AA, Kunze-Schumacher H, Blasczyk R, Bade-Döding C. Physiology and Pathology of Drug Hypersensitivity: Role of Human Leukocyte Antigens. In: Rezaei DN, editor. Physiology and Pathology of Immunology: InTech; 2017.

[11] Edwards IR, Aronson JK. Adverse drug reactions: definitions, diagnosis, and management. Lancet. 2000;356(9237):1255-1259.

[12] Ponnusankar S, Tejaswini M, Chaitanya M. Assessment of Adverse Drug Reactions Based on Spontaneous Signals at Secondary Care Public Hospital. Indian J Pharm Sci. 2015;77(4):490-493.

[13] Rawlins MD. Clinical pharmacology. Adverse reactions to drugs. British medical journal. 1981;282(6268):974-976.

[14] Pichler WJ, Hausmann O. Classification of Drug Hypersensitivity into Allergic, p-i, and Pseudo-Allergic Forms. International archives of allergy and immunology. 2016;171(3-4):166-179.

[15] Davies EC, Green CF, Taylor S, Williamson PR, Mottram DR, Pirmohamed M. Adverse drug reactions in hospital in-patients: a prospective analysis of 3695 patient-episodes. PloS one. 2009;4(2):e4439.

[16] Uetrecht J, Naisbitt DJ. Idiosyncratic adverse drug reactions: current concepts. Pharmacological reviews. 2013;65(2):779-808.

[17] Pirmohamed M, James S, Meakin S, Green C, Scott AK, Walley TJ, et al. Adverse drug reactions as cause of

admission to hospital: prospective analysis of 18 820 patients. Bmj. 2004;329(7456):15-19.

[18] Mittmann N, Knowles SR, Gomez M, Fish JS, Cartotto R, Shear NH. Evaluation of the extent of under-reporting of serious adverse drug reactions: the case of toxic epidermal necrolysis. Drug safety. 2004;27(7):477-487.

[19] Backstrom M, Mjorndal T, Dahlqvist R. Under-reporting of serious adverse drug reactions in Sweden. Pharmacoepidemiology and drug safety. 2004;13(7):483-487.

[20] Evans RS, Pestotnik SL, Classen DC, Bass SB, Burke JP. Prevention of adverse drug events through computerized surveillance. Proc Annu Symp Comput Appl Med Care. 1992:437-441.

[21] Simper GS, Graser LS, Celik AA, Kuhn J, Kunze-Schumacher H, Ho GT, et al. The Mechanistic Differences in HLA-Associated Carbamazepine Hypersensitivity. Pharmaceutics. 2019;11(10).

[22] McCormack M, Alfirevic A, Bourgeois S, Farrell JJ, Kasperaviciute D, Carrington M, et al. HLA-A*3101 and carbamazepine-induced hypersensitivity reactions in Europeans. The New England journal of medicine. 2011;364(12):1134-1143.

[23] Sidoroff A, Dunant A, Viboud C, Halevy S, Bavinck JN, Naldi L, et al. Risk factors for acute generalized exanthematous pustulosis (AGEP)-results of a multinational case-control study (EuroSCAR). The British journal of dermatology. 2007;157(5):989-996.

[24] Kardaun SH, Sekula P, Valeyrie-Allanore L, Liss Y, Chu CY, Creamer D, et al. Drug reaction with eosinophilia and systemic symptoms (DRESS): an original multisystem adverse drug reaction. Results from the prospective RegiSCAR study. The British journal of dermatology. 2013;169(5):1071-1080.

[25] Mockenhaupt M. Stevens-Johnson syndrome and toxic epidermal necrolysis: clinical patterns, diagnostic considerations, etiology, and therapeutic management. Semin Cutan Med Surg. 2014;33(1):10-16.

[26] Demoly P, Adkinson NF, Brockow K, Castells M, Chiriac AM, Greenberger PA, et al. International Consensus on drug allergy. Allergy. 2014;69(4):420-437.

[27] Yang Y, Li F, Du J, Shen Y, Lin J, Zhu X, et al. Variable levels of apoptotic signal-associated cytokines in the disease course of patients with Stevens-Johnson syndrome and toxic epidermal necrolysis. Australas J Dermatol. 2017;58(3):e61-ee7.

[28] Mockenhaupt M. The current understanding of Stevens-Johnson syndrome and toxic epidermal necrolysis. Expert review of clinical immunology. 2011;7(6):803-813; quiz 14-5.

[29] Sassolas B, Haddad C, Mockenhaupt M, Dunant A, Liss Y, Bork K, et al. ALDEN, an algorithm for assessment of drug causality in Stevens-Johnson Syndrome and toxic epidermal necrolysis: comparison with case-control analysis. Clinical pharmacology and therapeutics. 2010;88(1):60-68.

[30] Mockenhaupt M, Viboud C, Dunant A, Naldi L, Halevy S, Bouwes Bavinck JN, et al. Stevens-Johnson syndrome and toxic epidermal necrolysis: assessment of medication risks with emphasis on recently marketed drugs. The EuroSCAR-study. The Journal of investigative dermatology. 2008;128(1):35-44.

[31] Pirmohamed M, Ostrov DA, Park BK. New genetic findings lead the

way to a better understanding of fundamental mechanisms of drug hypersensitivity. The Journal of allergy and clinical immunology. 2015;136(2):236-244.

[32] Klein J, Sato A. The HLA system. First of two parts. The New England journal of medicine. 2000;343(10):702-709.

[33] York IA, Rock KL. Antigen processing and presentation by the class I major histocompatibility complex. Annual review of immunology. 1996;14:369-396.

[34] Chapman LM, Aggrey AA, Field DJ, Srivastava K, Ture S, Yui K, et al. Platelets present antigen in the context of MHC class I. Journal of immunology. 2012;189(2):916-923.

[35] Robinson J, Halliwell JA, Hayhurst JD, Flicek P, Parham P, Marsh SG. The IPD and IMGT/HLA database: allele variant databases. Nucleic acids research. 2015;43(Database issue):D423–D431.

[36] Klein J, Sato A. Birth of the major histocompatibility complex. Scandinavian journal of immunology. 1998;47(3):199-209.

[37] Mallal S, Nolan D, Witt C, Masel G, Martin AM, Moore C, et al. Association between presence of HLA-B*5701, HLA-DR7, and HLA-DQ3 and hypersensitivity to HIV-1 reverse-transcriptase inhibitor abacavir. Lancet. 2002;359(9308):727-732.

[38] Hetherington S, McGuirk S, Powell G, Cutrell A, Naderer O, Spreen B, et al. Hypersensitivity reactions during therapy with the nucleoside reverse transcriptase inhibitor abacavir. Clinical therapeutics. 2001;23(10):1603-1614.

[39] Mallal S, Phillips E, Carosi G, Molina JM, Workman C, Tomazic J, et al. HLA-B*5701 screening for hypersensitivity to abacavir. The New England journal of medicine. 2008;358(6):568-579.

[40] Hung SI, Chung WH, Liou LB, Chu CC, Lin M, Huang HP, et al. HLA-B*5801 allele as a genetic marker for severe cutaneous adverse reactions caused by allopurinol. Proceedings of the National Academy of Sciences of the United States of America. 2005;102(11):4134-4139.

[41] Chung WH, Hung SI, Hong HS, Hsih MS, Yang LC, Ho HC, et al. Medical genetics: a marker for Stevens-Johnson syndrome. Nature. 2004;428(6982):486.

[42] Hirata K, Takagi H, Yamamoto M, Matsumoto T, Nishiya T, Mori K, et al. Ticlopidine-induced hepatotoxicity is associated with specific human leukocyte antigen genomic subtypes in Japanese patients: a preliminary case-control study. The pharmacogenomics journal. 2008;8(1):29-33.

[43] Zhang FR, Liu H, Irwanto A, Fu XA, Li Y, Yu GQ, et al. HLA-B*13:01 and the dapsone hypersensitivity syndrome. The New England journal of medicine. 2013;369(17):1620-1628.

[44] Martin AM, Nolan D, James I, Cameron P, Keller J, Moore C, et al. Predisposition to nevirapine hypersensitivity associated with HLA-DRB1*0101 and abrogated by low CD4 T-cell counts. Aids. 2005;19(1):97-99.

[45] Hetherington S, Hughes AR, Mosteller M, Shortino D, Baker KL, Spreen W, et al. Genetic variations in HLA-B region and hypersensitivity reactions to abacavir. Lancet. 2002;359(9312):1121-1122.

[46] Hung SI, Chung WH, Jee SH, Chen WC, Chang YT, Lee WR, et al. Genetic susceptibility to carbamazepine-induced cutaneous adverse drug

reactions. Pharmacogenetics and genomics. 2006;16(4):297-306.

[47] Man CB, Kwan P, Baum L, Yu E, Lau KM, Cheng AS, et al. Association between HLA-B*1502 allele and antiepileptic drug-induced cutaneous reactions in Han Chinese. Epilepsia. 2007;48(5):1015-1018.

[48] Lonjou C, Borot N, Sekula P, Ledger N, Thomas L, Halevy S, et al. A European study of HLA-B in Stevens-Johnson syndrome and toxic epidermal necrolysis related to five high-risk drugs. Pharmacogenetics and genomics. 2008;18(2):99-107.

[49] Daly AK, Donaldson PT, Bhatnagar P, Shen Y, Pe'er I, Floratos A, et al. HLA-B*5701 genotype is a major determinant of drug-induced liver injury due to flucloxacillin. Nature genetics. 2009;41(7):816-819.

[50] Kazeem GR, Cox C, Aponte J, Messenheimer J, Brazell C, Nelsen AC, et al. High-resolution HLA genotyping and severe cutaneous adverse reactions in lamotrigine-treated patients. Pharmacogenetics and genomics. 2009;19(9):661-665.

[51] Hung SI, Chung WH, Liu ZS, Chen CH, Hsih MS, Hui RC, et al. Common risk allele in aromatic antiepileptic-drug induced Stevens-Johnson syndrome and toxic epidermal necrolysis in Han Chinese. Pharmacogenomics. 2010;11(3):349-356.

[52] Miguel A, Azevedo LF, Araujo M, Pereira AC. Frequency of adverse drug reactions in hospitalized patients: a systematic review and meta-analysis. Pharmacoepidemiology and drug safety. 2012;21(11):1139-1154.

[53] Solda T, Galli C, Kaufman RJ, Molinari M. Substrate-specific requirements for UGT1-dependent release from calnexin. Molecular cell. 2007;27(2):238-249.

[54] Sadasivan B, Lehner PJ, Ortmann B, Spies T, Cresswell P. Roles for calreticulin and a novel glycoprotein, tapasin, in the interaction of MHC class I molecules with TAP. Immunity. 1996;5(2):103-114.

[55] Strehl B, Seifert U, Kruger E, Heink S, Kuckelkorn U, Kloetzel PM. Interferon-gamma, the functional plasticity of the ubiquitin-proteasome system, and MHC class I antigen processing. Immunological reviews. 2005;207:19-30.

[56] Reits EA, Vos JC, Gromme M, Neefjes J. The major substrates for TAP in vivo are derived from newly synthesized proteins. Nature. 2000;404(6779):774-778.

[57] Schubert U, Anton LC, Gibbs J, Norbury CC, Yewdell JW, Bennink JR. Rapid degradation of a large fraction of newly synthesized proteins by proteasomes. Nature. 2000;404(6779):770-774.

[58] Yewdell JW, Reits E, Neefjes J. Making sense of mass destruction: quantitating MHC class I antigen presentation. Nature reviews Immunology. 2003;3(12):952-961.

[59] Garrett TP, Saper MA, Bjorkman PJ, Strominger JL, Wiley DC. Specificity pockets for the side chains of peptide antigens in HLA-Aw68. Nature. 1989;342(6250):692-696.

[60] Madden DR. The three-dimensional structure of peptide-MHC complexes. Annual review of immunology. 1995;13:587-622.

[61] Huyton T, Ladas N, Schumacher H, Blasczyk R, Bade-Doeding C. Pocketcheck: updating the HLA class I peptide specificity roadmap. Tissue antigens. 2012;80(3):239-248.

[62] Wang R, Natarajan K, Margulies DH. Structural basis of the

CD8 alpha beta/MHC class I interaction: focused recognition orients CD8 beta to a T cell proximal position. Journal of immunology. 2009;183(4):2554-2564.

[63] Palacios EH, Weiss A. Function of the Src-family kinases, Lck and Fyn, in T-cell development and activation. Oncogene. 2004;23(48):7990-8000.

[64] Yasukawa M, Ohminami H, Arai J, Kasahara Y, Ishida Y, Fujita S. Granule exocytosis, and not the fas/fas ligand system, is the main pathway of cytotoxicity mediated by alloantigen-specific CD4(+) as well as CD8(+) cytotoxic T lymphocytes in humans. Blood. 2000;95(7):2352-2355.

[65] Le Cleach L, Delaire S, Boumsell L, Bagot M, Bourgault-Villada I, Bensussan A, et al. Blister fluid T lymphocytes during toxic epidermal necrolysis are functional cytotoxic cells which express human natural killer (NK) inhibitory receptors. Clinical and experimental immunology. 2000;119(1):225-230.

[66] Morel E, Alvarez L, Cabanas R, Fiandor A, Diaz R, Escamochero S, et al. Expression of alpha-defensin 1-3 in T cells from severe cutaneous drug-induced hypersensitivity reactions. Allergy. 2011;66(3):360-367.

[67] Landsteiner K, Jacobs J. Studies on the Sensitization of Animals with Simple Chemical Compounds. The Journal of experimental medicine. 1935;61(5):643-656.

[68] Gell PG, Harington CR, Rivers RP. The antigenic function of simple chemical compounds; production of precipitins in rabbits. British journal of experimental pathology. 1946;27(5):267-286.

[69] Eisen HN, Orris L, Belman S. Elicitation of delayed allergic skin reactions with haptens; the dependence of elicitation on hapten combination with protein. The Journal of experimental medicine. 1952;95(5):473-487.

[70] Park BK, Coleman JW, Kitteringham NR. Drug disposition and drug hypersensitivity. Biochemical pharmacology. 1987;36(5):581-590.

[71] Faulkner L, Meng X, Park BK, Naisbitt DJ. The importance of hapten-protein complex formation in the development of drug allergy. Current opinion in allergy and clinical immunology. 2014;14(4):293-300.

[72] Brander C, Mauri-Hellweg D, Bettens F, Rolli H, Goldman M, Pichler WJ. Heterogeneous T cell responses to beta-lactam-modified self-structures are observed in penicillin-allergic individuals. Journal of immunology. 1995;155(5):2670-2678.

[73] Schneider CH, De Weck AL. A new chemical spect of penicillin allergy: the direct reaction of penicillin with epsilon-amino-groups. Nature. 1965;208(5005):57-59.

[74] Padovan E, Mauri-Hellweg D, Pichler WJ, Weltzien HU. T cell recognition of penicillin G: structural features determining antigenic specificity. European journal of immunology. 1996;26(1):42-48.

[75] Romano A, Blanca M, Torres MJ, Bircher A, Aberer W, Brockow K, et al. Diagnosis of nonimmediate reactions to beta-lactam antibiotics. Allergy. 2004;59(11):1153-1160.

[76] Naisbitt DJ, Farrell J, Gordon SF, Maggs JL, Burkhart C, Pichler WJ, et al. Covalent binding of the nitroso metabolite of sulfamethoxazole leads to toxicity and major histocompatibility complex-restricted antigen presentation. Molecular pharmacology. 2002;62(3):628-637.

[77] Pichler WJ, Beeler A, Keller M, Lerch M, Posadas S, Schmid D, et al. Pharmacological interaction of drugs with immune receptors: the p-i concept. Allergology international : official journal of the Japanese Society of Allergology. 2006;55(1):17-25.

[78] Pichler WJ. The p-i Concept: Pharmacological Interaction of Drugs With Immune Receptors. The World Allergy Organization journal. 2008;1(6):96-102.

[79] Schnyder B, Mauri-Hellweg D, Zanni M, Bettens F, Pichler WJ. Direct, MHC-dependent presentation of the drug sulfamethoxazole to human alphabeta T cell clones. The Journal of clinical investigation. 1997;100(1):136-141.

[80] Pichler WJ. Delayed drug hypersensitivity reactions. Annals of internal medicine. 2003;139(8):683-693.

[81] Simper GS, Ho GT, Celik AA, Huyton T, Kuhn J, Kunze-Schumacher H, et al. Carbamazepine-Mediated Adverse Drug Reactions: CBZ-10,11-epoxide but Not Carbamazepine Induces the Alteration of Peptides Presented by HLA-B *15:02. Journal of immunology research. 2018;2018:5086503.

[82] Ostrov DA, Grant BJ, Pompeu YA, Sidney J, Harndahl M, Southwood S, et al. Drug hypersensitivity caused by alteration of the MHC-presented self-peptide repertoire. Proceedings of the National Academy of Sciences of the United States of America. 2012;109(25):9959-9964.

[83] Illing PT, Vivian JP, Dudek NL, Kostenko L, Chen Z, Bharadwaj M, et al. Immune self-reactivity triggered by drug-modified HLA-peptide repertoire. Nature. 2012;486(7404):554-558.

[84] Norcross MA, Luo S, Lu L, Boyne MT, Gomarteli M, Rennels AD, et al. Abacavir induces loading of novel self-peptides into HLA-B*57: 01: an autoimmune model for HLA-associated drug hypersensitivity. Aids. 2012;26(11):F21–F29.

[85] Shorvon SD. Drug treatment of epilepsy in the century of the ILAE: the second 50 years, 1959-2009. Epilepsia. 2009;50 Suppl 3:93-130.

[86] Gayford JJ, Redpath TH. The side-effects of carbamazepine. Proceedings of the Royal Society of Medicine. 1969;62(6):615-616.

[87] Schindler W HF. Über Derivate des Iminodibenzyls. Helvetica Chimica Acta 1954;37:472-483.

[88] Blom S. Trigeminal neuralgia: its treatment with a new anticonvulsant drug (G-32883). Lancet. 1962;1(7234): 839-840.

[89] Simpson JR. "Collagen disease" due to carbamazepine (Tegretol). British medical journal. 1966;2(5527):1434.

[90] Locharernkul C, Loplumlert J, Limotai C, Korkij W, Desudchit T, Tongkobpetch S, et al. Carbamazepine and phenytoin induced Stevens-Johnson syndrome is associated with HLA-B*1502 allele in Thai population. Epilepsia. 2008;49(12):2087-2091.

[91] Mehta TY, Prajapati LM, Mittal B, Joshi CG, Sheth JJ, Patel DB, et al. Association of HLA-B*1502 allele and carbamazepine-induced Stevens-Johnson syndrome among Indians. Indian journal of dermatology, venereology and leprology. 2009;75(6):579-582.

[92] Chang CC, Too CL, Murad S, Hussein SH. Association of HLA-B*1502 allele with carbamazepine-induced toxic epidermal necrolysis and Stevens-Johnson syndrome in the multi-ethnic Malaysian population. International journal of dermatology. 2011;50(2): 221-224.

[93] Kim SH, Lee KW, Song WJ, Kim SH, Jee YK, Lee SM, et al. Carbamazepine-induced severe cutaneous adverse reactions and HLA genotypes in Koreans. Epilepsy research. 2011;97(1-2):190-197.

[94] Ozeki T, Mushiroda T, Yowang A, Takahashi A, Kubo M, Shirakata Y, et al. Genome-wide association study identifies HLA-A*3101 allele as a genetic risk factor for carbamazepine-induced cutaneous adverse drug reactions in Japanese population. Human molecular genetics. 2011;20(5):1034-1041.

[95] Yip VL, Pirmohamed M. The HLA-A*31:01 allele: influence on carbamazepine treatment. Pharmgenomics Pers Med. 2017;10:29-38.

[96] Alfirevic A, Jorgensen AL, Williamson PR, Chadwick DW, Park BK, Pirmohamed M. HLA-B locus in Caucasian patients with carbamazepine hypersensitivity. Pharmacogenomics. 2006;7(6):813-818.

[97] Illing PT, Vivian JP, Purcell AW, Rossjohn J, McCluskey J. Human leukocyte antigen-associated drug hypersensitivity. Current opinion in immunology. 2013;25(1):81-89.

[98] Yang CW, Hung SI, Juo CG, Lin YP, Fang WH, Lu IH, et al. HLA-B*1502-bound peptides: implications for the pathogenesis of carbamazepine-induced Stevens-Johnson syndrome. The Journal of allergy and clinical immunology. 2007;120(4):870-877.

[99] Wei CY, Chung WH, Huang HW, Chen YT, Hung SI. Direct interaction between HLA-B and carbamazepine activates T cells in patients with Stevens-Johnson syndrome. The Journal of allergy and clinical immunology. 2012;129(6):1562-1569 e5.

[100] He XJ, Jian LY, He XL, Tang M, Wu Y, Xu YY, et al. Association of ABCB1, CYP3A4, EPHX1, FAS, SCN1A, MICA, and BAG6 polymorphisms with the risk of carbamazepine-induced Stevens-Johnson syndrome/toxic epidermal necrolysis in Chinese Han patients with epilepsy. Epilepsia. 2014;55(8):1301-1306.

[101] Ko TM, Chung WH, Wei CY, Shih HY, Chen JK, Lin CH, et al. Shared and restricted T-cell receptor use is crucial for carbamazepine-induced Stevens-Johnson syndrome. The Journal of allergy and clinical immunology. 2011;128(6):1266-1276 e11.

[102] Mizutani S, Pauwels E, Stoven V, Goto S, Yamanishi Y. Relating drug-protein interaction network with drug side effects. Bioinformatics. 2012;28(18):i522-i5i8.

[103] Schirle M, Bantscheff M, Kuster B. Mass spectrometry-based proteomics in preclinical drug discovery. Chem Biol. 2012;19(1):72-84.

[104] Hayes SA, Clarke S, Pavlakis N, Howell VM. The role of proteomics in the age of immunotherapies. Mamm Genome. 2018;29(11-12):757-769.

[105] Redwood AJ, Pavlos RK, White KD, Phillips EJ. HLAs: Key regulators of T-cell-mediated drug hypersensitivity. Hla. 2018;91(1):3-16.

Section 3

Drug Safety among Older People

Chapter 7

Pharmacovigilance in Older Adults

Daniel Gomes, Eva Rebelo Gomes, Inês Ribeiro-Vaz, Maria Teresa Herdeiro and Fátima Roque

Abstract

Polypharmacy and physiological changes inherent to the aging process can cause significant modifications in the pharmacokinetic and dynamic regimens of drugs, making the elderly more susceptible to adverse drug effects. Adverse drug reactions (ADR) in older adults have a significant impact on hospital admissions, increasing hospital stay and healthcare costs. Most common ADR in this population are dose-related and predictable. However, they can be difficult to diagnose as they often have nonspecific symptoms. This could be minimized by decreasing the use and prescription of potentially inappropriate medication and being aware of possible drug interactions. Besides, being older patients underrepresented in clinical trials and due to their physiological modifications, serious or atypical ADR are more common in this age range. To minimize harm in older adults, effective pharmacovigilance must be encouraged.

Keywords: Elderly, Medication, Adverse Drug Reactions, Drug Safety, Pharmacovigilance

1. Introduction

The World Health Organization [WHO] estimates that more than half of medicines are either inappropriately prescribed, dispensed, or sold, as the vast majority of patients fail to take their medication properly [1]. Adding the fact that no drug, taken correctly, is completely risk-free, it becomes of the outmost importance to permanently monitor its safety, to ensure that, throughout its life cycle, the benefits of each drug outweigh the risks of its use [2]. Pharmacovigilance intends to promote patient care and safety as well as an effective assessment of the risk–benefit profile of drugs [3].

With declining fertility rates and greater and better access to health care, the population aged, and the number of older adults has increased globally [4].

Aging is a risk factor for the development of chronic diseases, and to an increased incidence of pathologies such as cardiovascular diseases, strokes, cancer, or dementias. In this sense, the older population is the age group that most needs health care and medicines [5, 6]. Polypharmacy, commonly defined as the concomitant use of at least five drugs, is thus prevalent in this age group [7, 8].

Associated with aging, pharmacodynamic and pharmacokinetic changes occur at physiological level, which implies modified pharmacological responses [9]. The older are much more susceptible to adverse reactions and drug interactions than any other age group [7, 8].

Since people aged 65 and older are underrepresented in clinical trials pharmacovigilance becomes essential to allow continuous monitoring of safety and the assessment of the benefit/risk of drugs in this population [10].

2. Physiological and pharmacological modifications

The impact of aging on the human organism brings together complex changes at the molecular, cellular and tissue levels in all systems of the organism, and the effects of the most varied existing environmental factors [11, 12].

The physiological changes associated with the aging process weaken the older population. These can cause significant changes in the pharmacokinetic and dynamic regimens of medications, making them more susceptible to adverse effects [13].

2.1 Age-related changes in pharmacokinetics

With aging, pharmacokinetics processes suffer modifications [9]. Bioavailability, the extent and rate at which the active substance enters the systemic circulation to reach the action site, can be modified [9, 14].

Absorption of most drugs does not appear to decrease significantly with age, but different pathologies of the digestive system may affect drug absorption [9]. Nevertheless, drugs administered intramuscularly or subcutaneously may have their absorption modified, due to the reduction in blood perfusion of the tissues [15].

After absorption, the drug enters the bloodstream and is distributed to different tissues and organs. With the increase in fat mass and reduction in the volume of water, the volume of distribution of fat-soluble medications increases [as does the half-life of the same], as in the case for the long-acting benzodiazepines [15, 16]. In contrast, water-soluble drugs may have a lower volume of distribution, with an increase in plasma concentrations, that can be toxic, as happens with gentamicin, digoxin, theophylline, and cimetidine [9, 16]. In addition to body composition, the two main proteins involved in the transport of drugs: albumin, which binds to acidic drugs [e.g. warfarin, digoxin, lorazepam], and α1-acid glycoprotein, which binds mainly to basic drugs [ex: lidocaine, propranolol] may have their plasma concentrations altered in older population with comorbidities [15, 17].

Although other organs can metabolize drugs, the liver is the main organ involved in the process. Metabolism consists of converting an active substance in simpler and more polar substances, called metabolites, from phase I and II reactions. These metabolites are inactive or have modified activity. In the liver, maintaining its functions during aging, there are changes that can reduce its functionality [18]. The hepatic volume decreases 20–30%, and the hepatic blood flow 20–50%. There is a reduction in the first-pass hepatic effect, and thus the bioavailability of drugs that are subjected to extensive first-pass metabolism may be increased, while others, which need activation in the liver, may be reduced [15]. In addition, the hepatic clearance of drugs subjected to limited flow metabolism [e.g., propranolol and amitriptyline] can be reduced by more than 40%. Age can significantly affect the pharmacokinetics of drugs with a narrow therapeutic index [reduced margin between an effective dose and a toxic dose]. Inflammatory conditions can also affect the function of the enzymes involved in metabolism. The microbial ecosystem also stands out, with many clinically relevant drugs being co-metabolized by microflora. With changes in the composition of the intestinal microbiome, the drug's metabolism can also be altered with harmful consequences [19].

Excretion is also affected by the aging process. The kidney is the main organ in the removal of drugs and their metabolites and the pharmacokinetics are strongly influenced by the progressive loss of kidney function with age, thereby decreasing the excretion of drugs [20, 21]. Due to these changes, a decline in total clearance with age is expected for drugs predominantly excreted by this pathway. With the decrease in clearance, serum levels will increase, potentially causing ADR [22]. Therefore, the dosage of these drugs must be guided by kidney function and the glomerular filtration rate [GFR]. In addition, polypharmacy can increase the risk of kidney dysfunction, overloading the kidneys to excrete several drugs and their metabolites at the same time [23].

2.2 Age-related changes in pharmacodynamics

In older adults' sensitivity, meaning the effects of the same concentration of a particular drug at the site of action, vary significantly when comparing with young or adult persons. This difference can be justified by changes in drug-receptor interaction, signal transduction, adaptive homeostatic responses and, among more fragile patients, by comorbidities [24, 25]. Although age-related pharmacokinetic changes are predictable, the complex interaction between pharmacokinetic changes and homeostatic changes makes it a difficult topic to study [15].

The most relevant pharmacodynamic changes are at the central nervous system [CNS] and cardiovascular level [15]. Older adults often demonstrate an exaggerated response to psychoactive drugs due to an underlying age-related decline in CNS function, and are also more prone to adverse effects with cognitive impairment, including confusion and drowsiness. At the cardiovascular level, they may experience a greater decline in blood pressure after administration of calcium channel blockers with or without dihydropyridine, which may be the result of related changes with age in the reflex of the baroreceptors, as well as a decreased clearance of these drugs [25, 26]. In addition, β-adrenergic receptors decrease in numbers and have less sensitivity and also show changes in the G-protein involved in signal transduction. As a result, β-adrenergic activity in vascular, cardiac and respiratory tissue decreases, altering the effect of β-blocking agents and β-agonists in general [26, 27].

Pharmacodynamics not only affects the therapeutic effects of the drug but can also change the magnitude of the effect with subsequent adverse effects [20, 25]. These changes in pharmacokinetics and pharmacodynamics can thus make the older population more prone and susceptible to ADRs, either in normal therapeutic doses or by drug interactions mechanisms [27].

3. Adverse drug reactions in older adults

As previous mentioned, physiological aging causes pharmacodynamic and pharmacokinetic changes, imposing different pharmacological responses [9]. The drug could trigger iatrogenic problems in the geriatric patient, increasing the risk of possible ADR [28].

The vast majority of ADRs can be divided in 2 types:

- Dose-dependent, more frequent at higher doses, which can occur in any individual when exposed to a sufficient dose of the drug: Type A - Augmented, representing almost 80% of all ADR in older patients [29, 30]

- Immune mediated or non-immunological hypersensitivity reactions, not dependent on the dose, which can occur in predisposed individual. These reactions are therefore unpredictable and more serious, usually detected only after the drug enters the market: Type B - Bizarre, representing 20% of all ADRs in older patients [29–32].

Drugs associated with type A reactions are generally of low therapeutic index and are commonly used in older patients and therefore most ADRs in this age group are type A reactions with predictable pharmacological effect [30, 33]. Known homeostatic dysregulation, age-related changes in pharmacokinetics and pharmacodynamics and drug interactions make ADRs definitely or possibly preventable in this population. However, ADRs can be difficult to diagnose in older patients as they often have nonspecific symptoms, whether falls, fatigue, cognitive decline, or constipation, all of which have different etiologies [7]. Despite the difficulties it is estimated an average prevalence of 11% of ADR [33].

Most common ADRs causing hospitalization in older patients are related to Gastrointestinal complications [Gastrointestinal bleeding, peptic ulcer, erosive gastritis, nausea, vomiting]; Cardiovascular disorders [Hypotension, bradycardia, falls, arrhythmias] Metabolic/endocrine complications [Hypoglycemia]; Renal and urinary disorders [Renal impairment, acute renal failure]; Electrolyte disorders [Hypokalemia, hyperkalemia, hyponatremia]; Nervous system disorders [Depressed level of consciousness, mental status changes] [34]. Studies have shown that beta-blockers, antibiotics, oral anticoagulants, digoxin, ACE inhibitors, antineoplastics, calcium entry blockers, opioids, oral antidiabetics and most frequently NSAIDs as the main drug classes causing ADR hospitalization in older adults [33, 35].

3.1 The healthcare impact of ADR in older patients

ADRs cause a significant burden in healthcare services, representing 6.5% in hospital admissions, being responsible for death of 0.15% of the patients admitted. Besides, patients admitted with ADRs were significantly older than patients without ADRs, as hospitalization due to NSAIDs complications increases exponentially with aging, having an important impact in healthcare resources. The median prevalence of ADRs leading to hospitalization is 10%. Although some hospitalizations related to ADRs are inevitable, it is estimated that only 18.6–28% of ADR cases that caused hospitalization in older patients were considered inevitable. Severe ADRs are related mostly to hematological disorders and acute renal failure [33, 34].

Polypharmacy is one of the main risk factors for ADR in this population. The risk of ADR increases by 13% in patients taking two drugs to 58% when taking five and to 82% when taking seven or more drugs [4, 7]. Drug interactions, common in polypharmacy, can cause synergistic toxicity and thus be risk factors, such as the combination of corticosteroids and NSAIDs. Polypharmacy leads to problems in medication adherence and correct administration representing a risk for adverse events or ADR [31, 36, 37].

ADRs also have a strong economic impact in the health system. The costs involved in treatment are mainly associated with hospitalization, prolonged hospital stay and additional clinical investigations- Studies point to an average of 8 additional hospital stay days and costs of approximately 706 M € per year [38, 39]. Regarding avoidable ADRs, costs per hospitalization vary between € 2,851 - 9,015, with length of hospital stay between 4.2 and 13 days. In outpatient, the costs resulting from avoidable ADRs ranged between € 174 and € 8,515 [38]. Particularly in the elderly, an average cost of emergency care of 333 US $ is pointed, with severe ADR patients costing $ 691 per patient and $ 7,529 per patient with severe ADR during hospitalization [40].

ADRs can trigger cascades of prescription when new drugs are prescribed for problems resulting from another medication, which is usually an unknown ADR, increasing therapeutic costs, in addition to increasing the risk of new ADRs. Fever, hemorrhage, diarrhea and arrhythmia are those with the greatest economic burden in a hospital environment; and NSAIDs, antibiotics, anticoagulants and antineoplastics are the main classes involved in ADRs related costs [39].

Most drugs are suitable for the older, as long as they are used in the correct dose and for the necessary period. However, since they are more susceptible to adverse events, the potential risk of certain drugs may outweigh the potential benefit. When safer alternatives are available, these drugs are considered inappropriate [PIM] [28, 41].

3.2 Potentially inappropriate medication for older adults

In recent years, in order to reduce inappropriate prescribing, and in turn, to reduce the prevalence of PIM in older population, explicit and implicit criteria strategies and tools have been developed, being very useful in clinical practice, as decision support- Explicit criteria consists in lists of drugs applied with minimal information and clinical evaluation, not considering individual differences between patients, representing important alert mechanisms on the possibility of the inappropriate use of a medication just by itself, as where implicit criteria focus on the patient's therapeutic regimen and clinical evaluation. Associating these criteria with information management tools such as Clinical decision support systems [CDSS] can allow improvements in patient therapy. These CSSDs, usually computerized, can verify interactions between medicine-disease or medicine-medicine, also detecting PIM [36].

Among the criteria most applied in research within this theme, Beers criteria stands out. In 1991, Beers and his research colleagues met with geriatric and pharmaceutical specialists to list the drugs to be avoided by older people. Explicit criteria were defined, considering 30 drugs/pharmacological groups considered inappropriate. These criteria have since been repeatedly reformulated and updated according to new information in the literature. Currently, these criteria are divided into 5 lists: Potentially inappropriate to be avoided in the elderly; Potentially inappropriate in the elderly due to drug–drug and/or drug-disease interactions; Those that should be prescribed with caution in the elderly; Combinations of drugs known to cause "drug–drug" interactions; Drugs to be avoided or whose dose adjustment is necessary when prescribed in elderly people with impaired renal function [42, 43]. However, its application in Europe is limited, where several of the drugs identified in these criteria are not commercialized in this continent and some of the drugs marketed in Europe are inappropriate and are not on the Beers list [44].

START/ STOPP criteria is also currently used. The STOPP [Screening Tool of Older Person's potentially inappropriate Prescriptions] criteria are 80 parameters organized by physiological systems. The START [Screening Tool to Alert doctors to Right Treatment], on the other hand, identify potentially beneficial omissions [which should be prescribed to the elderly], with 34 criteria divided into six physiological systems [44]. STOPP/START have advantages over Beers because they are significantly associated with adverse drug reactions. In addition, they are more in line with the European reality, also having greater sensitivity demonstrated for the identification of inappropriate prescriptions. Although the STOPP criteria is explicit, only 29 of the 81 STOPP criteria can be applied only with information on the patient's medication profile [36].

Recently, in order to develop a European list of potentially inappropriate drugs, 27 experts from 7 countries in Europe came together, creating the EU [7] -PIM list, with

282 drugs from 34 pharmacological classes in which it is found, for each drug, the justification for its inadequacy, as well as dose adjustments/special considerations of use [when applicable] and possible alternatives to that drug [45].

The EU [7]-PIM list has been used in some studies in Europe that show a range between 40.9 [Sweden] and 87% [Portugal] of older adults having PIM prescribed by the physician. Proton bomb inhibitors, Bromazepam, Diazepam, Lorazepam and Alprazolam are the most common [46].

ADRs related to PIMs were observed in some studies, with digoxin, benzodiazepines, and imipraminic antidepressants, being the most common. In hospitalized older patients, NSAIDs were the most common types of PIM-ADRs, inducing upper gastrointestinal bleeding. Benzodiazepines inducing falls with fractures and depressed mental status, as well as digoxin >0.125 mg/day inducing cardiac arrhythmias and visual disturbances due to digoxin poisoning are also common in hospital context [47, 48].

4. Promoting drug safety in older adults

Older adults have a higher chronic diseases burden and consume more prescription drugs than any other age group. Besides drug–drug interactions, the prevalence of concurrent use of prescription drugs and herbal medicinal products [HMPs] by older adults is significant, and can also lead to serious ADR, as risk of bleeding due to the use concomitant use of *Ginkgo biloba*, garlic or ginseng with antithrombotics [49].

4.1 Older participants in clinical trials

Including older patients in the clinical trial process is important, as on average older adults carry 60% of the national disease burden but represent only 32% of participants in Phase II and III clinical trials [50, 51]. This population is underrepresented, especially the >75-year-old. and current guidelines recommend to have a significant number of older participants in the trials [that can be estimated with the help of epidemiological studies targeting the disease that the drug intends to treat] in order to assess the risk–benefit ratio of the drug in this age group. Phase I trials might not need older participants, but phase II and III clinical trials should include them, to assess dosage, safety, adverse effects, and effectiveness [52, 53]. Decentralized clinical trials could facilitate the appropriate inclusion of these patients [50].

Nevertheless, including this age group implies some methodological considerations. As it exists a progressive impairment of the renal or hepatic function or drug–drug interactions, an appropriate assessment of pharmacokinetic profiles and pharmacodynamic endpoints are needed [54, 55]. Besides, since they have a high risk of cognitive function impairment, determining adverse CNS events is of the outmost relevant clinical importance during the trial design. Aware of these needs, the International Council for Harmonization of Technical Requirements for Pharmaceuticals for Human Use [ICH] developed guidelines for studies in special populations, namely older adults, aiming for a sufficient representation in phase III. It is advisable 100 minimum participants and, when the disease is associated with aging, older people should form most of the participants [55, 56].

These studies should compare older and younger patients or evaluate drug disease interaction studies in older adults. Population pharmacokinetic analyses intends to determine the sources and correlation of variability of the drug concentration in the target patient population, comparing the older with the young group.

Safety and efficacy should also be of the outmost importance, as outcomes must be explored to provide evidence base support to the dose selection during drug approval, impacting regulatory procedures. Finding significant differences in safety and efficacy outcomes between young and older patients, pharmacokinetic studies plays an important role to understand these differences and assess benefit–risk of a drug administration [55–57].

4.2 Medication labelling

After drug development, providing quality information to health care professionals about the safe and effective use of drugs in geriatric patients is fundamental. And so, it is required by the Food and Drug Administration [FDA] and the European Medicines Agency [EMA] that the labeling of these drugs must have safety and efficacy information for the older. Particularly for EMA, it is mandatory to present on the Summary of Product Characteristics [SmPC] and the Patient Information Leaflet information regarding dosage, frequency and seriousness of ADR, or the need of monitoring in this population [57, 58].

4.3 Pharmacovigilance in older patients

Pharmacovigilance plays a key role in ADR detection in post authorization period, improving the safe and rational drug use and thereby improving patient care [59, 52]. In 2012, new legislation came into force within EU, creating the Pharmacovigilance Risk Assessment Committee and giving a central role to pharmacovigilance. A significant increase in the participation of health professionals and patients in the system was seen, and the electronic transmission of information from Pharmacovigilance became mandatory in November 2005, with EudraVigilance being the system for analyzing and managing information on suspected ADR, allowing the electronic exchange of reports of ADR cases, used by the various partners of the European regulatory network to monitor the safety of medicines [60].

A strong pharmacovigilance system can perform safety surveillance with processes, tools, and experts to monitor ADRs from medication taken by older patients. During this post-authorization surveillance, safety risks may be detected, particularly in patients with comorbidity and polypharmacy, suffering physiologic changes inherent to the aging process [61, 62]. Adequate pharmacovigilance systems considering HMPs is also necessary to increase the likelihood of ADR detection, and appropriately identify and manage older patients at risk [49, 63].

Risk management plans [RMP] must also be submitted to EMA when applying for a marketing authorization, including relevant information on medicine's safety profile, how the risks will be prevented or minimized and how to promote knowledge regarding safety and efficacy of a determined drug.. The elaboration of this document allows the understanding of safety concerns in older adults, planning how to reduce the possibility of suffering ADR. The RMP must be modified whenever it is determined important safety risks, as well as the labeling [54, 64].

Nevertheless, signal detection using spontaneous reporting systems is one of the most important sources for safety monitoring in post authorization "real-life" setting, especially in populations underrepresented in preapproval clinical trials such as older adults [61, 62]. Even tough underreporting, low sensitivity and selectivity are disadvantages to be considered regarding this reporting system, the fact that broadens all medicines on the market throughout all the life cycle, in all patients, not interfering with prescription habits, not only allows the identification of common ADR, as well as rare, unexpected ADRs in groups and scenarios not studied, as the older patients. This makes spontaneous reporting a fundamental report system for the safety monitoring of approved medicines [60, 65]. Due to the widespread of under-reporting of ADRs to spontaneous reporting systems, including serious or severe ADRs, the use of new technology is a great opportunity to empower patients to report, such as the programmes WEB-RADR [66] in Europe and Medwatch [67] in the United States. Although these tools were developed to facilitate reporting by both healthcare professionals and patients, a better understanding of the relation that the older patients have with health technologies is need [68].

In the European Economic Area [EEA], the electronic transmission of information from Pharmacovigilance became mandatory in November 2005, with EudraVigilance being the system for analyzing and managing information on suspected ADR, facilitating electronic exchange of individual case safety reports between EMA, national competent authorities, marketing authorization holders and sponsors of clinical trials in the EEA, as it allows early detection and evaluation of possible safety signals [60, 69].

EudraVigilance allows researchers and/or interested readers to perform same analysis in the ADR database EudraVigilance of the EMA, even though with different levels of access for different stakeholders. As some studies explore national databases, some studies have explored EudraVigilance database, accessing suspected medication and common ADR reported in older adults. Antineoplastic and immunomodulating agents, Nervous system, Cardiovascular system, Blood, and blood forming organs represent a significant part of suspected medication spontaneously reported in elderly. Rash, Confusional state, Dizziness, Pruritus, Pyrexia, Thrombocytopenia, Diarrhea, Vomiting, Dyspnea and Nausea are the most reported Preferred Terms in elderly spontaneous cases [62, 70, 71].

5. Conclusions

Older adults, having comorbidities, in polypharmacy regimens, associated with physiological age-related changes, are more susceptible to ADRs. With the demographic aging being a reality worldwide, the healthcare demand increases, as well as drug safety vigilance efforts.

Only recently older people start to have a significant presence in clinical trials. Pharmaceutical companies and the regulatory agencies joined efforts to provide evidence on the benefits and harms of medicines in older patients, giving more importance to efficacy and safety during drug development targeting diseases mostly related with aging or chronic diseases.

Pharmacovigilance regulatory agencies at a local and national level should promote monitoring and reporting programs of adverse effects observed, particularly in older populations, adding reliable safety data and identifying age related.

Drug safety studies in this age group need to be constantly improved to present evidence-based data to enhance quality of prescriptions in a highly healthcare demanding age group.

Acknowledgements

This work was financially supported by the project APIMedOlder [PTDC/MED-FAR/31598/2017], funded by FEDER, through COMPETE2020 – Programa Operacional Competitividade e Internacionalização [POCI-01-0145-FEDER-031598], and by national funds [OE], through FCT/MCTES. Replace the entirety of this text with acknowledgments.

Conflict of interest

The authors declare no conflict of interest.

Appendices and Nomenclature

ADR	Adverse drug reaction
CDSS	Clinical decision support systems
CNS	Central nervous system
EEA	European Economic Area
EMA	European Medicines Agency
FDA	Food and Drug Administration
GFR	Glomerular Filtration Rate
ICH	International Council for Harmonization of Technical Requirements for Pharmaceuticals for Human Use
NSAID	Non-steroid anti-inflammatory drug
RMP	Risk Management Plan
SmPC	Summary of Product Characteristics
WHO	World Health Organization

Author details

Daniel Gomes[1,2], Eva Rebelo Gomes[3], Inês Ribeiro-Vaz[4,5], Maria Teresa Herdeiro[6] and Fátima Roque[1,7]*

1 Research Unit for Inland Development, Polytechnic of Guarda (UDI-IPG), Guarda, Portugal

2 Faculty of Economics, University of Coimbra (FFUC), Coimbra, Portugal

3 Allergy and Clinical Immunology Service, University Hospital Center of Porto, Porto, Portugal

4 Porto Pharmacovigilance Centre, Faculty of Medicine, University of Porto, Portugal

5 Center for Health Technology and Services Research (CINTESIS), Faculty of Medicine, University of Porto, Portugal

6 Department of Medical Sciences, Institute of Biomedicine, University of Aveiro (iBIMED-UA), Aveiro, Portugal

7 Health Sciences Research Centre, University of Beira Interior (CICS-UBI), Covilhã, Portugal

*Address all correspondence to: froque@ipg.pt

References

[1] World Health Organization. The Pursuit of Responsible Use of Medicines: Sharing and Learning from Country Experiences The benefits of responsible use of medicines: Setting policies for better and cost-effective health care [Internet]. 2012 [cited 2020 Nov 29]. Available from: www.who.int

[2] FDA. Think It Through: Managing the Benefits and Risks of Medicines | FDA [Internet]. [cited 2020 Nov 29]. Available from: https://www.fda.gov/drugs/drug-information-consumers/think-it-through-managing-benefits-and-risks-medicines

[3] UMC | The story of UMC and the WHO programme [Internet]. [cited 2020 Nov 30]. Available from: https://www.who-umc.org/global-pharmacovigilance/who-programme-for-international-drug-monitoring/the-story-of-umc-and-the-who-programme/

[4] World Health Organization. Global Health and Aging. Global Health and Aging. 2011.

[5] Atella V, Mortari AP, Kopinska J, Federico Belotti |, Lapi F, Cricelli C, et al. Trends in age-related disease burden and healthcare utilization. Aging Cell. 2018;

[6] Santos M, Almeida A. Polimedicação no Idoso. Rev Enferm Ref. 2010;III[n°2].

[7] Lavan AH, Gallagher P. Predicting risk of adverse drug reactions in older adults. Ther Adv Drug Saf. 2016;

[8] WHO. Medication Safety in Polypharmacy. Geneva; 2019.

[9] Mangoni AA, Jackson SHD. Age-related changes in pharmacokinetics and pharmacodynamics: basic principles and practical applications. Br J Clin Pharmacol [Internet]. 2004;57[1]:6-14. Available from: http://www.ncbi.nlm.nih.gov/pubmed/14678335%0Ahttp://www.pubmedcentral.nih.gov/articlerender.fcgi?artid=PMC1884408

[10] Jose J. Promoting drug safety in elderly - Needs a proactive approach [Internet]. Vol. 136, Indian Journal of Medical Research. Wolters Kluwer -- Medknow Publications; 2012 [cited 2020 Nov 30]. p. 362-4. Available from: https://www.ncbi.nlm.nih.gov/pmc/articles/PMC3510880/

[11] Kriete A, Sokhansanj BA, Coppock DL, West GB. Systems approaches to the networks of aging. Vol. 5, Ageing Research Reviews. Ageing Res Rev; 2006. p. 434-448.

[12] Maguire SL, Slater BMJ. Physiology of ageing. Vol. 11, Anaesthesia and Intensive Care Medicine. Elsevier Ltd; 2010. p. 290-292.

[13] Koren G, Nordon G, Radinsky K, Shalev V. Clinical pharmacology of old age. Vol. 12, Expert Review of Clinical Pharmacology. Taylor and Francis Ltd; 2019. p. 749-55.

[14] MSD Manual Professional Edition. Drug Bioavailability - Clinical Pharmacology. 2019.

[15] Corsonello A, Pedone C, Incalzi R. Age-Related Pharmacokinetic and Pharmacodynamic Changes and Related Risk of Adverse Drug Reactions. Curr Med Chem. 2010 Jan;17[6]:571-584.

[16] Hämmerlein A, Derendorf H, Lowenthal DT. Pharmacokinetic and pharmacodynamic changes in the elderly. Clinical implications. Vol. 35, Clinical Pharmacokinetics. 1998. p. 49-64.

[17] Bteich M. An overview of albumin and alpha-1-acid glycoprotein main characteristics: highlighting the roles of

amino acids in binding kinetics and molecular interactions. Heliyon. 2017;e02879.

[18] Shi S, Klotz U. Age-Related Changes in Pharmacokinetics. Curr Drug Metab. 2011 Jul;12[7]:601-610.

[19] Waring RH, Harris RM, Mitchell SC. Drug metabolism in the elderly: A multifactorial problem? Vol. 100, Maturitas. Elsevier Ireland Ltd; 2017. p. 27-32.

[20] Aymanns C, Keller F, Maus S, Hartmann B, Czock D. Review on pharmacokinetics and pharmacodynamics and the aging kidney. Clin J Am Soc Nephrol. 2010;5[2]:314-327.

[21] Reeve E, Wiese MD, Mangoni AA. Alterations in drug disposition in older adults. Vol. 11, Expert Opinion on Drug Metabolism and Toxicology. Informa Healthcare; 2015. p. 491-508.

[22] Turnheim K. When drug therapy gets old: Pharmacokinetics and pharmacodynamics in the elderly. Exp Gerontol. 2003;38[8]:843-853.

[23] Kang H, Hong SH. Risk of Kidney Dysfunction from Polypharmacy among Older Patients: A Nested Case-Control Study of the South Korean Senior Cohort. Sci Rep. 2019;9[1]:1-11.

[24] Ruscin JM, Linnebur SA. Pharmacodynamics in Older Adults . 2018.

[25] Sera L, Uritsky T. Pharmacokinetic and pharmacodynamic changes in older adults and implications for palliative care. Prog Palliat Care. 2016 Sep;24[5]:255-261.

[26] Bowie MW, Slattum PW. Pharmacodynamics in Older Adults: A Review. Am J Geriatr Pharmacother. 2007 Sep;5[3]:263-303.

[27] Bressler R, Bahl JJ. Principles of Drug Therapy for the Elderly Patient. In: Mayo Clinic Proceedings. Elsevier Ltd; 2003. p. 1564-1577.

[28] Spinewine A, Schmader KE, Barber N, Hughes C, Lapane KL, Swine C, et al. Appropriate prescribing in elderly people: how well can it be measured and optimised? Vol. 370, Lancet. 2007. p. 173-184.

[29] Bowman L, Carlstedt BC, Hancock EF, Black CD. Adverse drug reaction [ADR] occurrence and evaluation in elderly inpatients. Pharmacoepidemiol Drug Saf [Internet]. 1996 Jan [cited 2020 Nov 30];5[1]:9-18. Available from: https://pubmed.ncbi.nlm.nih.gov/15088272/

[30] Kaufman G. Adverse drug reactions: classification, susceptibility and reporting. Nurs Stand. 2016;30[50]: 53-63.

[31] Brahma DK, Wahlang JB, Marak MD, Sangma MC. Adverse drug reactions in the elderly. J Pharmacol Pharmacother. 2013;4[2]:91-94.

[32] Management Sciences for Health, WHO. Drug and Therapeutics Committee Training Course. 2007.

[33] Alhawassi TM, Krass I, Bajorek B, Pont LG. A systematic review of the prevalence and risk factors for adverse drug reactions in the elderly in the acute care setting. Clin Interv Aging. 2014;9:2079-2086.

[34] Nair NP, Chalmers L, Peterson GM, Bereznicki BJ, Castelino RL, Bereznicki LR. Hospitalization in older patients due to adverse drug reactions - The need for a prediction tool. Clin Interv Aging. 2016;11:497-505.

[35] Oscanoa TJ, Lizaraso F, Carvajal A. Hospital admissions due to adverse drug reactions in the elderly. A meta-analysis.

Eur J Clin Pharmacol. 2017 Jun;73[6]:759-770.

[36] A. Rodrigues D, Teresa Herdeiro M, Figueiras A, Coutinho P, Roque F. Elderly and Polypharmacy: Physiological and Cognitive Changes. In: Frailty in the Elderly - Physical, Cognitive and Emotional Domains [Working Title]. IntechOpen; 2020.

[37] Gomes D, Placido AI, Mó R, Simões JL, Amaral O, Fernandes I, et al. Daily medication management and adherence in the polymedicated elderly: A cross-sectional study in Portugal. Int J Environ Res Public Health. 2020 Jan;17[1].

[38] Formica D, Sultana J, Cutroneo PM, Lucchesi S, Angelica R, Crisafulli S, et al. The economic burden of preventable adverse drug reactions: a systematic review of observational studies. Vol. 17, Expert Opinion on Drug Safety. Taylor and Francis Ltd; 2018. p. 681-95.

[39] Sultana J, Cutroneo P, Trifirò G. Clinical and economic burden of adverse drug reactions. Vol. 4, Journal of Pharmacology and Pharmacotherapeutics. Wolters Kluwer -- Medknow Publications; 2013. p. S73.

[40] Wu C, Bell CM, Wodchis WP. Incidence and Economic Burden of Adverse Drug Reactions among Elderly Patients in Ontario Emergency Departments. Drug Saf. 2012 Sep;35[9]:769-781.

[41] Pirmohamed M, James S, Meakin S, Green C, Scott AK, Walley TJ, et al. Adverse drug reactions as cause of admission to hospital: Prospective analysis of 18 820 patients. Br Med J [Internet]. 2004 Jul 3 [cited 2020 Nov 30];329[7456]:15-9. Available from: http://www.bmj.com/

[42] Beers MH, Ouslander JG, Rollingher I, Reuben DB, Brooks J, Beck JC. Explicit Criteria for Determining Inappropriate Medication Use in Nursing Home Residents. Arch Intern Med [Internet]. 1991 Sep 1 [cited 2020 Sep 6];151[9]:1825-32. Available from: https://jamanetwork.com/journals/jamainternalmedicine/fullarticle/615518

[43] Fick D, Semla T, Beizer J, Brandt N, Dombrowski R, DuBeau CE, et al. American Geriatrics Society updated Beers Criteria for potentially inappropriate medication use in older adults [Internet]. Vol. 60, Journal of the American Geriatrics Society. J Am Geriatr Soc; 2012 [cited 2020 Sep 6]. p. 616-31. Available from: https://pubmed.ncbi.nlm.nih.gov/22376048/

[44] Rei T, Ramôa A, Pereira C, Carvalho C, Fernandes C, Sousa LP, et al. Prescrição potencialmente inapropriada em idosos numa unidade de saúde familiar do norte do país – aplicação dos critérios stopp/start versão 2. AIMGF Mag. 2018;8[2].

[45] Renom-Guiteras A, Meyer G, Thürmann PA. The EU[7]-PIM list: a list of potentially inappropriate medications for older people consented by experts from seven European countries. Eur J Clin Pharmacol [Internet]. 2015 Jul 14 [cited 2020 Sep 18];71[7]:861-75. Available from: http://link.springer.com/10.1007/s00228-015-1860-9

[46] Rodrigues DA, Herdeiro MT, Thurmann PA, Figueiras A, Coutinho P, Roque F. Operacionalização para Portugal da Lista EU[7]-PIM para Identificação de Medicamentos Potencialmente Inapropriados nos Idosos Operationalisation for Portugal of the EU[7]-PIM List for Identification of Potentially Inappropriate Medicines in Older Adults. Acta Med Port [Internet]. 2020 Nov 23 [cited 2020 Nov 30];33[13]. Available from: www.actamedicaportuguesa.com

[47] Galli TB, Reis WCT, Andrzejevski VMS. Potentially

inappropriate prescribing and the risk of adverse drug reactions in critically ill older adults. Pharm Pract [Granada] [Internet]. 2016 Oct 1 [cited 2020 Nov 30];14[4]. Available from: /pmc/articles/PMC5184374/?report=abstract

[48] Montastruc F, Duguet C, Rousseau V, Bagheri H, Montastruc JL. Potentially inappropriate medications and adverse drug reactions in the elderly: A study in a PharmacoVigilance database. Eur J Clin Pharmacol [Internet]. 2014 [cited 2020 Nov 30];70[9]:1123-7. Available from: https://pubmed.ncbi.nlm.nih.gov/24925091/

[49] Agbabiaka TB, Wider B, Watson LK, Goodman C. Concurrent Use of Prescription Drugs and Herbal Medicinal Products in Older Adults: A Systematic Review [Internet]. Vol. 34, Drugs and Aging. Springer International Publishing; 2017 [cited 2020 Nov 30]. p. 891-905. Available from: /pmc/articles/PMC5730633/?report=abstract

[50] Guidance for including elderly patients in clinical trials | Cambridge Cognition [Internet]. [cited 2020 Nov 30]. Available from: https://www.cambridgecognition.com/blog/entry/guidance-for-including-elderly-patients-in-clinical-trials

[51] Montero D. Pharmacovigilance Pharmacovigilance and and the the elderly elderly Some Some proposals proposals for for improvement improvement.

[52] COMMITTEE FOR HUMAN MEDICINAL PRODUCTS. ADEQUACY OF GUIDANCE ON THE ELDERLY REGARDING MEDICINAL PRODUCTS FOR HUMAN USE [Internet]. 2012 [cited 2020 Nov 30]. Available from: http://www.emea.europa.eu

[53] Herrera AP, Snipes SA, King DW, Torres-Vigil I, Goldberg DS, Wenberg AD. Disparate inclusion of older adults in clinical trials: priorities and opportunities for policy and practice change. Am J Public Health [Internet]. 2010 Apr 1 [cited 2020 Nov 30];100[SUPPL. 1]:S105. Available from: /pmc/articles/PMC2837461/?report=abstract

[54] Medicines Agency E. Guideline on good pharmacovigilance practices [GVP] - Module VI – Collection, management and submission of reports of suspected adverse reactions to medicinal products [Rev 2] [Internet]. 2017 [cited 2020 Sep 20]. Available from: www.ema.europa.eu

[55] ICH. ICH Topic E7 Studies in Support of Special Populations: Geriatrics [Internet]. 1994 [cited 2020 Nov 30]. Available from: http://www.emea.eu.int

[56] FDA. Population Pharmacokinetics - Guidance for Industry [Internet]. 2019 [cited 2020 Nov 30]. Available from: https://www.fda.gov/Drugs/GuidanceComplianceRegulatoryInformation/Guidances/default.htm

[57] FDA. Guidance for Industry Content and Format for Geriatric Labeling [Internet]. 2001 [cited 2020 Nov 30]. Available from: http://www.fda.gov/cder/guidance/index.htm.or http://www.fda.gov/cber/guidelines.htm.Fax:1-888-CBERFAXor

[58] Malhotra R. Strategies for improving prescription medication labels for the elderly CARE Expert Programme | 3. 2017.

[59] World Health Organization. Regulation and Prequalification [Internet]. [cited 2020 Nov 30]. Available from: https://www.who.int/teams/regulation-prequalification/pharmacovigilance

[60] INFARMED I.P. Farma covigilância em Portugal: 25 anos. Oliveira Martins S, editor. 2019.

[61] Raine JM. Pharmacovigilance in the Elderly-highlights from informal PhVWP.

[62] Genov G. EudraVigilance and Signal Detection.

[63] Lima CMDS, Fujishima MAT, Santos BÉF Dos, Lima BDP, Mastroianni PC, Sousa FFO De, et al. Phytopharmacovigilance in the Elderly: Highlights from the Brazilian Amazon. Evidence-based Complement Altern Med [Internet]. 2019 [cited 2020 Nov 30];2019. Available from: /pmc/articles/PMC6378030/?report=abstract

[64] Risk management plans | European Medicines Agency [Internet]. [cited 2020 Nov 30]. Available from: https://www.ema.europa.eu/en/human-regulatory/marketing-authorisation/pharmacovigilance/risk-management/risk-management-plans

[65] Herdeiro MT, Ferreira M, Ribeiro-Vaz I, Junqueira Polónia J, Costa-Pereira A. O sistema Português de farmacovigilância. Acta Med Port. 2012;25[4]:241-249.

[66] WEB-RADR: Recognising Adverse Drug Reactions. [cited 2021 May 26]. Available from: https://web-radr.eu/

[67] MedWatch: The FDA Safety Information and Adverse Event Reporting Program. [cited 2021 May 26]. Available from: https://www.fda.gov/safety/medwatch-fda-safety-information-and-adverse-event-reporting-program.

[68] Etemad-Sajadi R, Gomes Dos Santos G. Senior citizens' acceptance of connected health technologies in their homes. J Health Care Qual Assur. 2019 Oct 14;32(8):1162-1174. doi: 10.1108/IJHCQA-10-2018-0240.

[69] EudraVigilance | European Medicines Agency [Internet]. [cited 2020 Nov 30]. Available from: https://www.ema.europa.eu/en/human-regulatory/research-development/pharmacovigilance/eudravigilance

[70] Monteiro C, Duarte AP, Alves G. Adverse drug reactions in elderly: a five-year review of spontaneous reports to the Portuguese Pharmacovigilance System. Expert Opin Drug Saf [Internet]. 2020 Nov 10 [cited 2020 Nov 30];14740338.2020.1849137. Available from: https://www.tandfonline.com/doi/full/10.1080/14740338.2020.1849137

[71] Dubrall D, Just KS, Schmid M, Stingl JC, Sachs B. Adverse drug reactions in older adults: A retrospective comparative analysis of spontaneous reports to the German Federal Institute for Drugs and Medical Devices. BMC Pharmacol Toxicol [Internet]. 2020 Mar 23 [cited 2020 Nov 30];21[1]:25. Available from: https://bmcpharmacoltoxicol.biomedcentral.com/articles/10.1186/s40360-020-0392-9

Chapter 8

Drug-Induced Delirium among Older People

Fabiana Rossi Varallo, Alan Maicon de Oliveira, Ariane Cristina Barboza Zanetti, Helaine Carneiro Capucho, Leonardo Régis Leira Pereira, Lucas Borges Pereira, Maria Olívia Barboza Zanetti, Thalita Zago Oliveira and Vinícius Detoni Lopes

Abstract

Although underdiagnosed, delirium is a common and potentially preventable problem in older patients, being associated with morbimortality. Drugs have been associated with the development of delirium in the geriatric population and may be considered the most easily reversible trigger. Polypharmacy, prescription of deliriogenic, anticholinergic and potentially inappropriate drugs are contributing factors for the occurrence of the disturb. Furthermore, changes in pharmacokinetic and pharmacodynamic parameters, which are intrinsic of the aged process, may contribute for cognitive impairment. Identification and reversal of clinical conditions associated with delirium are the first step to treat the disturbance, as well as mitigation of environmental factors and the exposition to deliriogenic drugs. Current evidence does not support the prescription of antipsychotics and benzodiazepines for the treatment of delirium. However, the judicious use of first- or second-generation antipsychotics can be considered in severe cases. Multi-component non-pharmacological, software-based intervention to identify medications that could contribute to delirium, predictive models, tools, training of health professionals and active actions of pharmacovigilance may contribute to the screening, prevention, and management of delirium in older people. Besides, it is also important to improve the report of drug-induced delirium in medical records, to develop properly risk management plans and avoid cascade iatrogenesis.

Keywords: aged, emergency service, hospital, drug-related side effects and adverse reactions, delirium, pharmacovigilance

1. Introduction

1.1 Definition, diagnosis and treatment

According to the Diagnostic and Statistical Manual of Mental Disorders [1], delirium is defined as a complex syndrome characterized by disturbance in attention (reduced ability to direct, focus, sustain, and shift attention), awareness (reduced orientation to the environment), and an additional disturbance in cognition (memory deficit, disorientation, language, visuospatial ability, or perception), which are not better explained by another preexisting, established, or evolving neurocognitive disorder. There is evidence that it is a direct physiological consequence of another medical condition, substance intoxication or withdrawal (i.e., due to a drug of abuse or to a medication), or exposure to a toxin, or is due to multiple etiologies [1]. The disturbance develops over a short period of time, usually from hours to a few days, and tends to fluctuate during the course of the day, often with worsening in the evening and night when external orienting stimuli decrease [1].

Delirium is considered a serious global public health problem because it can increase the rate of morbidity and mortality [2], prolong hospitalization, promote institutionalization, worsen physical, cognitive and social outcomes [3], besides to increase health costs [4] and loss of independence among people affected by this health condition [5].

Regarding clinical presentation of delirium based on the psychomotor behavior changes, delirium can be classified into: a) hyperactive (the individual has a hyperactive level of psychomotor activity that may be accompanied by mood lability, agitation, and/or refusal to cooperate with medical care); b) hypoactive (the individual has a hypoactive level of psychomotor activity that may be accompanied by sluggishness and lethargy that approaches stupor); c) mixed level of activity (the individual has a normal level of psychomotor activity even though attention and awareness are disturbed. It also includes individuals whose activity level rapidly fluctuates) [1]. Delirium can also be classified in 5 subtypes: i) substance intoxication delirium; ii) substance withdrawal delirium; iii) medication-induced delirium; iv) delirium due to another medical condition; and v) delirium due to multiple etiologies [1].

The diagnosis for medication-induced delirium is applied when disturbance in attention and an additional disturbance in cognition arise as an adverse drug reaction [1]. The codes for diagnoses, according to the 10th revision of the International Classification of Diseases and Related Health Problems (ICD-10), depend on the type of substance related to delirium (**Table 1**).

In June 2018, the World Health Organization (WHO) released a pre-final version of the ICD-11 [6]. Under mental, behavioral or neurodevelopmental disorders, the neurocognitive disorders group (6), includes delirium (6D70), which can also be classified as being due to: a medical condition classified elsewhere (6D70.0), psychoactive substances, including medications (6D70.1); multiple etiological factors (6D70.2), unknown or unspecified etiological factors (6D70.3), delirium, other specified cause (6D70.Y) and; delirium, unspecified or unknown cause (6D70.Z) [6].

Although the pathophysiological mechanisms of delirium remain unclear, several evidences suggest the participation of different neurotransmitters and biomarkers. Among the most investigated mechanisms is cholinergic dysfunction,

Substance	Withdrawal delirium	Intoxication delirium	ADR
Opioids	F11.231	F11.121; F11.221	F11.921
Sedative, hypnotic, or anxiolytic	F13.231	F13.121; F13.221	F13.921
Amphetamine (or other stimulant)	—	F15.121; F15.221	F15.921
Other classes	F19.231	F19.121; F19.221	F19.921

Legend: ADR = adverse drug reaction.
Source: DSM-5 (2013).

Table 1.
ICD-10-clinical modification codes for the [specific substance] related to delirium.

which may contribute to some of the manifestations known to be present in delirium, such as cognitive deficits associated with memory loss [7, 8].

Identification and reversal of clinical conditions associated with delirium are the first step to treat the disturbance, as well as mitigation of environmental factors and the exposure to deliriogenic drugs [9]. Non-pharmacological approaches should be provided in order to prevent and manage the neuropsychiatric symptoms related to delirium, such as: avoid the use of physical restraints, catheters, and bed alarms, ambulate patient, address sensory impairment, encourage exposure to bright light during the day, among others [8].

Current literature does not support the prescription of antipsychotics [10] and benzodiazepines [11] for the treatment of delirium in hospitalized patients. A meta-analysis study found that the prescription of antipsychotics did not control the symptoms of delirium nor reduced the severity and mortality associated with the disorder, when compared to other treatments. In addition, no differences were observed between typical and atypical antipsychotics in patients hospitalized in non-critical wards, regarding symptom resolution of delirium [12]. However, the judicious use of first- and second-generation antipsychotics can be considered for the treatment of severe delirium symptoms, especially in the management of agitation associated with the hyperactive subtype [13], as well as when non-pharmacological interventions have failed and the symptoms put the affected individual at risk and they are distressing for family and caregivers. In these cases, the treatment should start with low doses and be further titrated until the required effect is achieved [8].

Regarding prevention, multi-component non-pharmacological interventions have shown to reduce the incidence of delirium, compared to usual care adopted among non-critical inpatients [14]. However, there is no clear evidence that cholinesterase inhibitors, antipsychotic medication or melatonin is able to reduce its incidence [14]. Nevertheless, the use of technology to help pharmacist to identify medications associated with the occurrence of delirium may contribute to decrease the incidence of the disturbance in older people [15]. This approach allows for drug adjustments aiming to prevent or solve drug-related problems associated with neurological disorders.

2. Epidemiology of delirium

Delirium is the most common psychiatric syndrome in hospitalized patients [16]. The general occurrence of delirium cases in hospitals can be between 29 and 82%. In a systematic literature review, which assessed the occurrence of delirium in inpatients at the admission, the authors related an occurrence rate in Europe between 4% in France to 31% in Sweden [17]. In the community, this occurrence is reduced to 1–2%. This great difference in percentages results from the emergency units being the places where people presenting the signs and symptoms of delirium normally go to. In fact, 17% of the older people in the community and 40% of those who live in nursing homes frequently attend emergency units with this diagnosis. Moreover, during hospitalization there are many contributor factors for the increased risk of delirium occurrence [18, 19]. Therefore, differences in the incidence of delirium are observed among the different inpatient units within a hospital (**Table 2**). The intensive care units (ICU), palliative care, oncology and postoperative are usually the places where delirium events occur the most, around 50–82% [18, 19].

This wide variation in the occurrence of delirium, when comparing different units, can be extrapolated to its prognosis. The main prognoses in patients with delirium are falls, catheter-associated infection, weakness, longer hospital stay and death, with this risk being 2 to 4 times greater in patients admitted to the ICU, and

1.5 times greater in patients admitted to general wards [19]. For this reason, the prevention of delirium is very important in health care. Thus, improved knowledge of the main delirium-related risk factors is essential for all health professionals who assist these patients directly.

Although a single factor may cause delirium, especially in the older people, its occurrence is usually considered multifactorial. In addition, as noted in the incidence of cases, the occurrence of delirium is associated with patient's vulnerability to harmful factors, for example, critically ill patients may begin to experience delirium from the administration of a sedative, in contrast to healthy patients where this syndrome is unlikely to occur due to the involvement of a single stimulus. Consequently, there are individual-associated vulnerability factors, as well as precipitating factors that may potentially increase or not the risk of triggering delirium (**Table 3**) [18, 19].

	Incidence (%)
Surgical	
Cardiac	11–46
Non-cardiac	13–50
Orthopedic	12–51
Medical	
General medical	11–14
Old age medicine	20–29
Intensive care	19–82
Stroke	10–27
Dementia	56
Palliative care, cancer	47
Nursing home or post-acute care	20–22

Table 2.
Incidence of associated delirium in different inpatient units. Adapted from Inouye, 2014 [18].

Vulnerability factors of the individual	**Precipitating factors**
Age (> 70 years)	Polypharmacy (≥ 5 drugs)
Cognitive deficiency	Psychoactive use
Dementia	Infectious disease
Functional impairment	Surgery or trauma
Visual deficiency	Indwelling catheters
Stroke	Physical restrictions
History of alcohol dependence	Coma
Depression	Metabolic disorders (blood urea, abnormal pH values, sodium reduction, glucose reduction)
Multimorbidity	

Table 3.
Vulnerability factors of the individual and precipitating factors associated with the occurrence of delirium. Adapted from setters, 2017 [19].

In relation to the individual's vulnerability factors in the general population, the occurrence of delirium is normally more associated with involvement by other comorbidities, such as stroke and depression. In people admitted to hospitals, other factors are also associated with the occurrence of delirium, such as dementia, cognitive impairment, functional impairment, visual impairment, a history of high alcohol consumption, and advanced age (> 70 years) [18].

Regarding the precipitating factors, the occurrence of delirium in the general population is mostly associated with abnormal laboratory parameters, such as high serum urea. In inpatients, in addition to metabolic disorders resulting from laboratory tests, it is worth mentioning other important factors, such as polypharmacy (≥ 5 drugs), the use of psychoactive drugs, and especially physical restrictions [18].

3. Delirium in older people

Delirium is a common and potentially preventable syndrome in older people hospitalized patients, being associated with high mortality rates ranging from 25–33%, thus resulting in longer hospital stays, high health costs, functional decline, increased falls, hospital readmissions, development of dementia or long-term cognitive impairment, and higher rates of morbidity. Delirium can also cause adverse events after hospitalization, including lasting functional limitations, persistent cognitive decline, and loss of quality of life for the patient and caregivers. The occurrence of new cases of delirium during hospitalization of older people varies from 6–56%; while the prevalence of delirium at the time of admission of older people varies from 14–24%. Furthermore, with the population's advancing age, delirium stands as a public health concern as it tends to increase in the future [20–23].

Although in some cases delirium can be caused by a single drug or underlying disease, in most cases delirium is the result of the combined action of predisposing and precipitating factors. It is, therefore, a multifactorial condition, which involves the interrelation between the patient's vulnerability to delirium at the time of hospital admission (predisposing factors) and precipitating factors that may arise during hospitalization. In this perspective, patients considered vulnerable (for example, those with dementia or a serious underlying disease) may experience delirium due to the use of a single dose of a sedative aimed to sleep. In contrast, patients resistant to the development of delirium may present this condition after a series of combinations, such as general anesthesia, major surgery, sleep deprivation, immobilization and the use of multiple psychoactive drugs [20]. In general, an intervention in one or more of these factors is considered sufficient for the delirium to be resolved [23].

The main predisposing factors for the occurrence of delirium at the time of hospital admission are the severity of the underlying disease, visual deficit, basal cognitive level, and dehydration. On the other hand, there are precipitating factors contributing for the development of delirium during hospitalization, for example: use of physical restrictions, malnutrition, addition of more than three drugs in the previous day, especially psychoactive drugs, use of urinary catheter. It is known that dementia is the most prevalent predisposing factor at the time of hospital admission, since it is able to increase the possibility of developing delirium by two to five times; however, any chronic disease can predispose delirium. Among the precipitating factors, the use of drugs is emphasized, being considered an extremely usual factor during hospitalization, originating up to 40% of cases. Consequently, the occurrence of delirium increases in direct proportion to the number of drugs used, due to the greater chance of adverse events and drug interactions take place [23].

Thus, in order to prevent the development of delirium resulting from the use of drugs, it became necessary to develop risk management plans, which is currently a prerequisite for a good pharmacovigilance service [9].

It is a fact that the prevention of delirium in the older people should stand as the main goal throughout the health care supply provided by health professionals, since the delirium prevention is always preferable to its treatment. However, when delirium occurs, early intervention and adequate management have been shown to improve the results for these patients [21, 22]. Despite the adverse consequences associated with delirium, the performance of health professionals in recognizing, registering, and treating it is still inappropriate. The lack of knowledge of the risk factors related to delirium in hospitalized older people is responsible for failures in the records in medical charts, in the notification and in the communication of the occurrence of delirium. In addition, the existence of knowledge gaps in screening and diagnosis using evidence-based tools are the main barriers to care [22].

Confirming the diagnosis of delirium in older people can be a challenge in complex clinical situations, with multiple demands and even more when the diagnosis is made by non-specialized health centers or unskilled professionals. The clinical manifestations of delirium and the factors associated with this condition can be confused with elements characteristic of aging, as well as being recognized as only cases of dementia or depression [24, 25]. The assessment of delirium superimposed on pre-existing dementia must be part of the differential diagnosis, as it happens in 90% of the cases with hospitalized older people [26]. In addition, hyperactive presentations of delirium can be misdiagnosed as hypomanic episodes [24, 25]. Estimates indicate that the recognition of delirium in the usual care only happens in 12–35% of the occurrences [26].

Considering that the prevention of delirium is essential in health institutions, clinical guidelines and models promoting the prevention, diagnosis and treatment of delirium have been developed and published internationally. However, it appears that they have not been properly implemented in clinical practice, which reinforces the need to initiate patient-centered care approach in the detection, prevention, and treatment of delirium, as well as in discharge planning [27].

The prediction of delirium in health services is extremely relevant to direct resources to prevention programs for patients most likely to have the syndrome. Although different tools have been developed in recent years, there are still no predictive models with adequate performance and recommendations for routine use in health services. Considering the current period of evidence, the insertion of predictive modeling and artificial intelligence in the health sector is a promising field for future research [28]. Moreover, when associated with a patient safety program, it has the potential to significantly improve the quality of care.

To improve this scenario, there are support strategies and tools for the delirium evaluation. Initially, it is extremely important to be aware of the signs and symptoms, as well as in the early observation of their onset (appearance of disorders and mental fluctuations), to avoid undesirable worsening [18, 26]. Therefore, the history of the episode is fundamental, with the record consistency of the steps that resulted in the event and thus it will be possible to carry out a comprehensive assessment of the potential triggering causes [18, 26]. Thus, the notoriety of providing instruction for people is justified because, in addition to the health team, family members and/or caregivers will also be crucial for the collection of this information [18].

Regarding the diagnostic decision support tools, studies in the literature have shown to provide validated instruments for this purpose [29]. Among them, it is worth highlighting the Confusion Assessment Method (CAM) [30], due to the reliability of its psychometric properties (specificity of 89% and sensitivity of 94%)

and because of the amount of evidence supporting the improvements in the evaluation resulting from its use [18, 31].

Acute beginning, confused thinking, lack of concentration, impaired consciousness, disorientation, noticeable disorders, hypoactivity and hyperactivity, detriment of memory and alteration of the sleep–wake cycle are the factors analyzed by CAM, with an application time of 5 minutes [30]. Still on the applicability, this tool has versions adapted to the areas that differ in the levels of health care for the older people (nursing home, emergency and intensive care units) [32, 33]. In order to guarantee the sensitivity and specificity of the CAM, there is an indication for the rater to be trained for the timely administration of the method and, to ensure the hypothesis of delirium, the older people's cognition should be evaluated by some specific test (for example, Short Portable Mental Status Questionnaire [34], Mini-Mental State Examination [35], Montreal Cognitive Assessment [36] or the Mini-Cog [37]).

The Confusion Assessment Method (CAM) Diagnostic Algorithm [30].

- **Feature 1: Acute onset and fluctuating course**

  This feature is usually obtained from a reliable reporter, such as a family member, caregiver, or nurse, and is shown by positive responses to the questions: Is there evidence of an acute change in mental status from the patient's baseline? Did the (abnormal) behavior fluctuate during the day, that is, tend to come and go, or did it increase or decrease in severity?

- **Feature 2: Inattention**

  This feature is demonstrated by a positive response to the question: Did the patient have difficulty focusing attention, for example, being easily distractible, or have difficulty keeping track of what was being said?

- **Feature 3: Disorganized thinking**

  This feature is shown by a positive response to the question: Was the patient's thinking disorganized or incoherent, such as rambling or irrelevant conversation, unclear or illogical flow of ideas, or unpredictable switching from subject to subject?

- **Feature 4: Altered level of consciousness**

  This feature is demonstrated by any answer other than "alert" to the question: Overall, how would you rate this patient's level of consciousness? (alert [normal], vigilant [hyperalert], lethargic [drowsy, easily aroused], stupor [difficult to arouse], or coma [unarousable]).

The diagnosis of delirium by CAM requires the presence of features 1 and 2 and either 3 or 4.

However, the implementation of delirium screening, detection, documentation, and notification guidelines present several challenges, being associated with a series of contextual and organizational issues. One of the major issues to be considered by health professionals is the use of a variety of descriptors to document and communicate their delirium assessments, since important and necessary information for the prevention and treatment of delirium may not be efficiently communicated in the medical records [22].

Medical records generally include descriptors, such as disorientation, agitation, altered level of consciousness, fluctuating mental state, confusion, negative behavior and hallucinations, but the term delirium is rarely mentioned [22]. This factor restricts the identification of this type of incident in an active pharmacovigilance system, as well as impairs the proper assessment of the case in the process of passive surveillance of drug-related adverse events. Therefore, it is essential to take into consideration on these evidence-based techniques, given that episodes of delirium are related to geriatric syndromes (incontinence, pressure injuries and falls), and with a long-term prognosis of attenuated survival rate, health conditions that result in the need for rehabilitation and other adversities that affect cognition, such as dementia [18, 38]. Older people who were affected by delirium can be stratified in a public vulnerable to poor outcomes and this context predicts an alarming epidemic, given the increase in population longevity [38].

The Agency for Healthcare Research and Quality (AHRQ) points out delirium as an indicator of healthcare quality, because it is estimated that up to 40% of cases can be avoided in the general population and preventive interventions must involve the care environment (for example, lighting, availability of calendar, clock and other signages), the culture of team practices (for example, implementation of protocols for screening and continuous assessment of delirium, deprescribing and review of pharmacotherapy), in addition to measures for preliminary identification of risk factors [39]. Preventing, recognizing, and treating delirium has become a public health priority.

Owing to achieve quality and safety attributes at all levels of care for the older people, in addition of taking into account the severity of the complications caused (as poor quality of life, increased hospital stay and risk of death) and the high consecutive costs (from $ 143 to $ 152 billion per year), it is necessary to encourage the training of health professionals enabling them to recognize cases of delirium, as well as risk factors, treatment and prevention [18, 26]. The adequate documentation concerning the occurrence of delirium in health services and the initiative to educate the population about this disorder, can greatly contribute to the improvements in the management of this clinical condition [18, 26].

4. Drug related problems (DRPs) in the context of drug-induced delirium

Older people are a population at high risk for presenting DRPs and unnecessarily suffer from diseases and injuries resulting from excessive or inadequate consumption of drugs. Drug-induced delirium appears as a frequent consequence of these DRPs, which are associated with aspects of necessity, adherence, effectiveness, or safety of pharmacological treatment. In the care of older patients, the regular review of the pharmacotherapy is an essential service, but it is often neglected. Hospital and community pharmacists are in an ideal position to perform this task [40].

The behavior of the health professional team in just renewing previous prescriptions of polymedicated patients, without practicing review of pharmacotherapy, may result in the maintenance of treatments that are no longer necessary. Thereby, it becomes essential to assess the maintenance of each drug in terms of its benefit, when compared to the deliriogenic potential and the anticholinergic burden, with additional caution in drug discontinuation in those patients displaying an increased probability of delirium due to substance withdrawal syndrome [41]. The review should also include over-the-counter or easily accessible medications, herbal medicines and supplements, which are also associated with delirium (e.g. anticholinergics, antihistamines, non steroidal inflammatory drugs, muscle relaxants) [41, 42].

Any drug used to treat delirium, such as antipsychotics and benzodiazepines, will cause psychoactive effects and may further impair the state of consciousness. Therefore, the prescription of such drugs should be discouraged as they consist in a DRP of necessity (unnecessary drug), except in cases with severe symptoms that put the older people at risk, especially in the management of agitation associated with the hyperactive subtype of delirium. If the use of antipsychotics is indeed mandatory, the lowest dose and the shortest treatment period possible should be the chosen option. Benzodiazepines are restricted to the management of delirium due to alcohol and other drugs withdrawal [13, 43].

On the other hand, pharmacological treatment is regularly necessary in the management of factors that can contribute to the alteration of the state of consciousness, such as pain, infections, kidney disease, dehydration, metabolic and hydroelectrolytic disorders, among others [18, 19]. The absence of pharmacological interventions in this regard also constitutes a DRP (necessary drug not prescribed).

Delirium can also be a result of adherence problems (DRP of adherence). Aging brings a series of physical, mental, and social barriers to the adequate follow-up of pharmacotherapy, such as impaired vision, hearing and dexterity, difficulty in understanding and lack of home support. In the pharmacotherapeutic scheme, confusion predisposes to the occurrence of overdoses or even to the abrupt withdrawal of drugs, situations that trigger delirium. The pharmacist can develop strategies to make self-administration easier, aware the patient and reduce the complexity of pharmacotherapy (drug or formulation change, making boxes and guidelines, activation of alarms, etc.), in addition to educational actions for encouraging adherence [40, 44].

Some non-pharmacological factors can also contribute to the development of delirium and, when treated ineffectively (DRP of effectiveness), they may increase the chance of its occurrence. The sharp change in attention, awareness and cognitive functions can be triggered, for example, by uncontrolled infection, dehydration condition not reversed, and inadequate pain management (insufficient doses of opioids) [45].

All subtypes of delirium can be induced by Adverse Drug Reactions (ADR) [46]. When attention and cognition disturbance appear as a side effect of a drug taken as prescribed, this is characterized as a DRP of safety [1].

In older people, especially those diagnosed with dementia [46], most of these deliriogenic drugs have anticholinergic properties and are considered potentially inappropriate for this age group [47–49], with pyrilamine and methscopolamine being recently added to the list of drugs to be avoided [48].

Other drugs previously reported as capable of inducing delirium are opioids, antihypertensives (beta blockers associated with higher delirium rates when compared to calcium channel blockers), diuretics with the potential to cause hyponatremia, and dopaminergics [46, 50–52]. Abrupt withdrawal of benzodiazepines is related to hyperactive delirium, so de-escalation is advised [46].

Although the drugs described above are more often related to the development of delirium, it is essential to consider most drugs as risk factors in older people, due to the delirogenic potential of the aging process, illness or hospitalization [50]. Therefore, deprescribing should be considered when feasible.

In the case of drugs with anticholinergic activity, mainly muscarinic, changes in pharmacokinetic and pharmacodynamic parameters with advancing age increase the susceptibility to induce delirium [53]. After identifying those who potentiate delirium, they should be stopped or replaced by safer medicines [54].

Strategies for identifying, preventing, and solving actual and potential DRP essentially include the review of the pharmacotherapy and pharmacotherapeutic follow-up. These pharmaceutical services contribute to the prevention and resolution of deliriogenic drugs-induced ADR, decrease the incidence of delirium, minimize the occurrence of adverse events in people who are being treated with antipsychotics and allow polypharmacy to be assessed [55, 56].

5. Auxiliary instruments in the active search for DRPs in the context of drug-induced delirium

Most adverse events in the older people, especially those related to delirium, could be prevented by avoiding the prescription of Potentially Inappropriate

Medication (PIM), especially when safer alternatives are available for use. Most deliriogenic drugs have anticholinergic properties and are considered to be PIMs [47–49].

The development of evidence-based PIM lists is a complex task, as the geriatric population is usually excluded from clinical trials. Based on the opinion and consensus of experts, including pharmacists, geriatricians, nurses and other health professionals, several tools have been developed to assess whether drug use in the older people is appropriate [57]. One of the most used is the American Geriatrics Society (AGS) Beers Criteria, which was developed in the United States in 1991 and has further undergone several updates, the most recent one being published in 2019 [48]. The latest version of the AGS Beers Criteria organizes PIMs in five lists: drugs that are potentially inappropriate for the majority of the older people (high risk of adverse events and the existence of safer alternatives); drugs that should be avoided in older adults with specific clinical conditions; drugs to be used with caution; combinations of drugs that can cause harmful interactions; drugs that should be avoided or that require dose adjustment in the older people with impaired kidney function [48].

Another widely used prescription screening tool in the older people is the STOPP/START criteria, created in 2008 in Europe and updated in 2014 [58]. This tool is composed by the topics STOPP (Screening Tool of Older Persons' Prescriptions), which presents a list of PIMs organized by physiological systems, and START (Screening Tool to Alert to Right Treatment), which warns about missing treatments that should be initiated in older adults. This instrument also includes drug–drug interactions and drug-physiological status interactions [58].

Despite the existence of a large number of lists, tools and criteria for PIMs within the scientific literature, other factors should also be considered when reviewing pharmacotherapy, such as the older people's particularities, biological age, other therapeutic options and the specific needs of each patient.

The risk of drug-induced delirium in older adults can be assessed by the Delirium Drug Scale (DDS) [59]. The rank for the deliriogenic burden ranges from 0 to 3, according to the potential of the drug to induce delirium. Considering each drug with a potential delirium risk, the weighted DDS score should be calculated, so the exposure to the drugs that induce delirium is considered low when the scores vary between 0 and 1 excluding the value of 0; and high the score obtaind from DDS is greater than 1 [60]. Low exposure to drugs leading to delirium does not significantly increase the chances of delirium. For this reason, if the benefits of the therapy outweigh the risks, the prescribed doses can be safely tolerated [60].

Regarding the anticholinergic burden, the sum of the scores of anticholinergic activity magnitude for each prescribed drug, ranging from 1 to 3, is performed. The higher magnitude of anticholinergic activity leads to a higher score attributed to the drug [61]. Although there is no consensus in the literature, the average daily anticholinergic load ≥2 is considered high [62]. High anticholinergic burden is associated with increased risk of morbidity and mortality, hospital stay length, institutionalization, functional and cognitive decline [61].

6. Strategies for mitigating and preventing drug-induced delirium

6.1 Risk management: active and passive monitoring strategies for drug-related adverse events

Ensuring the safe use of drugs is one of the priorities of health systems worldwide, given that the estimated global cost due to failures in the process of using these technologies is approximately US $ 42 billion annually. The safety use of drugs is a complex concept comprising multifactorial origins in different stages of the prescription, dispensing and administration processes, and in all these processes there is a risk of drug-related adverse events, meaning, the harms that may arise from the inadequate/inappropriate use of these medicines [63].

The occurrence of drug-related adverse events is distinguished as a relevant cause of morbidity and mortality, by causing suffering and dissatisfaction of patients and rising health care costs [64]. Thus, it is important to use strategies to prevent the incidence of adverse events and to mitigate the resulting social and economic impacts.

Drug-related adverse events are the main cause of preventable harms to the patient, with monitoring strategies occurring through two types of surveillance systems: active and passive. In this context, in order to reduce incidents, including drug-related adverse events, many health systems have implemented passive surveillance systems, which are allusive to spontaneous incident reports, aiming to identify and describe the risks and causes associated with adverse events, harmless incidents and near misses [64]. As they are cost-effective, these voluntary notification systems are responsible for a large part of the reports containing drug-related adverse events, conferring the potential to improve health care through the monitoring, reduction, and prevention of adverse events. However, there are still challenges associated with the data obtained from these systems, as this information is often difficult to interpret and manipulate due to underreporting, as well as their content and variability in the attribution of event categories by notifiers [64, 65].

Therefore, active surveillance systems complement passive systems. Although the active system is more costly, the information is obtained through direct contact, at regular intervals, between the team responsible for the active search and intensive monitoring of adverse events and the sources of information, mainly through the analysis of documents linked to the medical records of the patients, either retrospectively or prospectively [64, 66].

6.2 Patient safety, pharmacovigilance, and delirium

Delirium is an indicator of health quality in older people and, therefore, its prevention is an essential parameter for patient safety. Given the association between delirium and other common geriatric syndromes, its prevention benefits the improvement of the quality and efficiency of health services. The prevalence of delirium, its severity and duration can be significantly reduced when considering the existing risk factors [67].

The current management of delirium emphasizes the importance of its prevention, preferably through a non-pharmacological approach implemented in multiple sectors of health services. In this context, the following actions for patient safety are highlighted as [56, 59, 67]:

- Staff training: health professionals involved in the care of patients should be trained in relation to delirium, its diagnosis, management, and adequate documentation;

- Support from health professionals in providing guidance on the environment: the hospital environment must be adapted to the special needs of patients. The decline in sensory function in older adults can cause additional psychosocial stress, which may be exacerbated by cognitive impairment. In these circumstances, appropriate signs can be placed in the patients' wards, rooms, and bathrooms. Tools for temporal and situational guidance can be made available, such as charts with personal information, date, and year, as well as clocks visible to patients. In addition, suitable accessories can be made available to prevent falls;

- Hospital admission phase: the health team can implement some non-pharmacological preventive interventions in this phase, for instance the realization of verbal guidelines, written recommendations for patients (posters, leaflets), instructions to the health team on the prescribed drugs and interventions and the appropriate ages;

- Implementation of treatments advised by international guidelines for the prevention of delirium: adaptation of surgeries and anesthesia; use of medications and pain treatment appropriate to the patient's age; pain monitoring; prevention of movement restrictions, such as when using catheters; use of benzodiazepines and anticholinergic drugs should be avoided; prescription of individualized and significant daily activities for the prevention of delirium, for example reorientation, cognitive activation, non-pharmacological promotion of sleep, and reduction of anxiety;

- Patients and their families should be individually advised on the risk and prevention of delirium. Family members can support individualized activities to prevent delirium by providing specific information about the patient, by collaborating with health care and by promoting individualized communication.

It is noteworthy that drug toxicity and polypharmacy are two of the main risk factors associated to delirium, especially in older patients with underlying comorbidities [62]. Anticholinergic, antipsychotic, benzodiazepine, and opioid agents are known to be highly deliriogenic [50]. However, several case reports show that drugs with a low suspicion of being deliriogenic can, in fact, present this particularity [68]. Therefore, the institutionalization of pharmacovigilance protocols for the management of delirium risks associated with the use of medications are of utmost importance.

The pharmacovigilance system is responsible for monitoring the safety of drugs and for adopting measures to reduce the risks and increase the benefits related to the use of drugs, as well as enabling improvements in patient safety and quality of life. Pharmacovigilance activities include: collecting and managing data on drug safety; the analysis of individual case reports to detect new drug-related adverse events; the proactive risk management to minimize any potential risks related to medication use; the communication and information to stakeholders and patients [69].

The suspected cases of delirium associated with the use of drugs identified by health service professionals, users and caregivers are notified to the drug manufacturers and health authorities in order to record these potential adverse events in the pharmacovigilance system. Such conduct makes it possible to screen and investigate the real association between these notified drugs and delirium. Notifications are generally sent voluntarily and reviewed by governmental organizations responsible for the safety of drugs on the market, which, in turn, forward the notifications to the Uppsala Monitoring Center, the World Health Organization collaborating centre for international drug monitoring.

For these reasons, it is highly important to establish a database to assess the safety issues of drugs in the post-marketing stage. This database system will allow to increase public knowledge regarding the drugs capable of inducing delirium, namely by identifying and monitoring the already known deliriogenic drugs, those potentially deliriogenic, as well as new drugs displaying the potential to cause delirium [68].

Finally, the knowledge regarding the frequency with which these potentially deliriogenic drugs are attributed as the primary cause of delirium has shown to help in the clinical practice and in the possible prevention of the [20]. Therefore, the elaboration of a list of drugs that are notably potentially deliriogenic and have the potential to cause delirium demands a plausibility research to determine a definitive association. This list of drugs associated with delirium can provide valuable information to health professionals, allowing for the prevention of delirium or its timely diagnosis, apart from avoiding other adverse events [68].

The knowledge about this important drug-related adverse event involving the occurrence of delirium can promote concrete actions to improve the quality of care for the older people, with the active participation of the multidisciplinary team, especially with a systematic implementation of institutional protocols for the prevention of delirium. Thus, it is essential to increase the population's knowledge, especially of health professionals, about delirium, its associated risks, and the need to document suspected cases of delirium associated with the use of drugs. Pharmacovigilance is the right tool for this.

7. Conclusions

In sum, delirium may increase morbidity and mortality, prolong the length of hospital stay, promote institutional long-term care, worsen functional, cognitive, and social outcomes, increase health costs, and exacerbate the loss of independence of older people. The most common factors significantly associated with delirium among this population are severity of medical illness, visual impairment, urinary catheterisation, electrolyte disturbance, immobility, frailty, and length of hospital stay. The use of deliriogenic, anticholinergic and potentially inappropriate drugs, as well polypharmacy, are also contributing factors to the occurrence of delirium.

To prevent the harm associated with acute cognitive impairment, pharmacovigilance activities, pharmaceutical care in the geriatric population and predictive models are advised, since they may contribute to the screening, prevention, and management of delirium. Furthermore, it is important to improve competences of healthcare professionals to properly report the occurrence of delirium in medical records and apply patient-centred clinical methods to prevent iatrogenic cascades.

Appendices and Nomenclature

ADR	Adverse Drug Reactions
AGS	American Geriatrics Society
AHRQ	Agency for Healthcare Research and Quality
CAM	Confusion Assessment Method
DDS	Delirium Drug Scale
DRPs	Drug Related Problems
ICD	International Classification of Diseases and Related Health Problems
ICU	intensive care unit
PIM	Potentially Inappropriate Medication
START	Screening Tool to Alert to Right Treatment
STOPP	Screening Tool of Older Persons' Prescriptions
WHO	World Health Organization

Author details

Fabiana Rossi Varallo[1*], Alan Maicon de Oliveira[1], Ariane Cristina Barboza Zanetti[1], Helaine Carneiro Capucho[2], Leonardo Régis Leira Pereira[1], Lucas Borges Pereira[1], Maria Olívia Barboza Zanetti[1], Thalita Zago Oliveira[1] and Vinícius Detoni Lopes[1]

1 School of Pharmaceutical Sciences of Ribeirao Preto, University of Sao Paulo, Ribeirão Preto (SP), Brazil

2 Pharmacy Department, University of Brasilia, Brasilia (DF), Brazil

*Address all correspondence to: frvarallo@fcfrp.usp.br

References

[1] APS. Diagnostic and Statistical Manual of Mental Disorders (DSM-5®) 5th Edition;2013.

[2] Dani M, Owen LH, Jackson TA, Rockwood K, Sampson EL, Davis D. Delirium, frailty, and mortality: interactions in a prospective study of hospitalized older people. J Gerontol a Biol Sci Med Sci. 2018;73(3):415-418.

[3] Minden SL, Carbone LA, Barsky A, Borus JF, Fife A, Fricchione GL, Orav EJ. Predictors and outcomes of delirium. Gen Hosp Psychiatry. 2005; 27(3):209-14.

[4] Leslie DL, Marcantonio ER, Zhang Y, Leo-Summers L, Ynouye SK. et al. One-year health care costs associated with delirium in the elderly population. Arch Intern Med 2008;168(1):27-32.

[5] Oh ES, Fong TG, Hshieh TT, Inouye SK. Delirium in older persons: advances in diagnosis and treatment. JAMA. 2017;318(12):1161-1174.

[6] World Health Organization. International Classification of Diseases for Mortality and Morbidity Statistics-Eleven Revision (11 ICD). Disposable at https://icd.who.int/browse11/l-m/en#/http://id.who.int/icd/entity/897917531. Accessed in November 20th, 2020

[7] Maldonado JR. Neuropathogenesis of delirium: review of current etiologic theories and common pathways. Am J Geriatr Psychiatry. 2013; 21(12): 1190-1222.

[8] Hshieh TH, Inouye SK, Oh ES Delirium in the Elderly. Clin Geriatr Med 2020; 36(2):183-19.

[9] Kassie GM, Ellett LMK, Nguyen TA, Roughead EE. Use of medicines that may precipitate delirium prior to hospitalisation in older Australians with delirium: An observational study. Australas J Ageing.; 2019; 38(2):124-131.

[10] Neufeld KJ, Yue J, Robinson TN, Inouye SK, Needham DM. Antipsychotic Medication for Prevention and Treatment of Delirium in Hospitalized Adults: A Systematic Review and Meta-Analysis. J Am Geriatr Soc. 2016;64(4):705-14.

[11] Li Y, Ma J, Jin Y, Li N, Zheng R. et al. Benzodiazepines for treatment of patients with delirium excluding those who are cared for in an intensive care unit. Cochrane Database Syst Rev. 2020; 2(2): CD012670.

[12] Burry L, Mehta S, Perreault MM, Luxenberg JS, Siddiqi N, Hutton B, Fergusson DA, Bell C, Rose L. Antipsychotics for treatment of delirium in hospitalised non- ICU patients (Review). Cochrane Database Syst Rev. 2018 ;6(6):CD005594.

[13] Han JH, Suyama J. Delirium and Dementia. Clinics in Geriatric Medicine; 2018; 34 (3): 327-354.

[14] Siddiqi N, Harrison JK, Clegg A, Teale EA, Young J, Taylor J, Simpkins SA. Interventions for preventing delirium in hospitalised non-ICU patients. Cochrane Database Syst Rev, 2016;3:CD005563.

[15] Woodhouse R, Burton JK, Rana N, Pang YL, Lister JE, Siddiqi N. Interventions for preventing delirium in older people in institutional long-term care. Cochrane Database Syst Rev; 2019;4(4):CD009537.

[16] Thom RP, Levy-Carrick NC, Phil M, Bui M, Silbersweig D. Delirium. Am J Psychiatry. 2019; 176:10. DOI: 10.1176/appi.ajp.2018.18070893.

[17] Siddiqi N, House AO, Holmes JD. Occurrence and outcome of delirium in medical in-inpatients: a systematic literature review. Age Ageing. 2006;35: 350-364. DOI: 10.1093/ageing/afl005.

[18] Inouye SK, Westendorp RG, Saczynski JS. Delirium in elderly people. Lancet. 2014 Mar 8;383(9920):911-22. doi: 10.1016/S0140-6736(13)60688-1

[19] Setters B, Solberg LM. Delirium. Prim Care Clin Office Pract. 2017; 44:541-559. DOI: 10.1016/j.pop.2017.04.010

[20] Inouye SK. Prevention of delirium in hospitalized older patients: Risk factors and targeted intervention strategies. Ann Med. 2000;32: 257-263. DOI:10.3109/07853890009011770

[21] Strijbos MJ, Steunenberg B, van der Mast RC, Inouye SK, Schuurmans MJ. Design and methods of the Hospital Elder Life Program (HELP), a multicomponent targeted intervention to prevent delirium in hospitalized older patients: efficacy and cost-effectiveness in Dutch health care. BMC Geriatr. 2013;13: 78. DOI:10.1186/1471-2318-13-78

[22] Zalon ML, Sandhaus S, Kovaleski M, Roe-Prior P. Hospitalized older adults with established delirium: Recognition, documentation, and reporting. J Gerontol Nurs. 2017;43: 32-40. DOI:10.3928/00989134-20161109-01

[23] Lôbo RR, Silva Filho SRB, Lima NKC, Ferriolli E, Moriguti JC. Delirium. Med (Ribeirao Preto Online). 2010;43: 249. DOI:10.11606/issn.2176-7262.v43i3p249-257

[24] Hall RJ, Meagher DJ, MacLullich AM. Delirium detection and monitoring outside the ICU. Best Pract Res Clin Anaesthesiol. 2012 Sep;26(3):367-83. DOI: 10.1016/j.bpa.2012.07.002

[25] Leonard M, Spiller J, Keen J, MacLullich A, Kamholtz B, Meagher D. Symptoms of depression and delirium assessed serially in palliative-care inpatients. Psychosomatics. 2009 Sep-Oct;50(5):506-14. doi: 10.1176/appi.psy.50.5.506.

[26] American Academy of Nursing. Twenty-Five Things Nurses and Patients Should Question. Choosing Wisely: an initiative of the ABIM Foundtion, 2018. Available from: https://www.choosingwisely.org/societies/american-academy-of-nursing/

[27] Lee-Steere K, Liddle J, Mudge A, Bennett S, McRae P, Barrimore SE. "You've got to keep moving, keep going": Understanding older patients' experiences and perceptions of delirium and nonpharmacological delirium prevention strategies in the acute hospital setting. J Clin Nurs. 2020;29: 2363-2377. DOI:10.1111/jocn.15248

[28] Rieck KM, Pagali S, Miller DM. Delirium in hospitalized older adults. Hospital practice (1995). NLM (Medline); 2020. pp. 3-16. DOI:10.1080/21548331.2019.1709359

[29] Adamis D, Sharma N, Whelan PJ, Macdonald AJ. Delirium scales: A review of current evidence. Aging Ment Health. 2010 Jul;14(5):543-55. doi: 10.1080/13607860903421011.

[30] Inouye SK, van Dyck CH, Alessi CA, Balkin S, Siegal AP, Horwitz RI. Clarifying confusion: the confusion assessment method. A new method for detection of delirium. Ann Intern Med. 1990 Dec 15;113(12):941-8. DOI: 10.7326/0003-4819-113-12-941

[31] Wong CL, Holroyd-Leduc J, Simel DL, Straus SE. Does this patient have delirium?: value of bedside instruments. JAMA. 2010 Aug 18;304(7):779-86. DOI: 10.1001/jama.2010.1182

[32] Han JH, Zimmerman EE, Cutler N, Schnelle J, Morandi A, Dittus RS, et al. Delirium in older emergency department patients: recognition, risk factors, and psychomotor subtypes. Acad Emerg Med. 2009 Mar;16(3):193-200. DOI: 10.1111/j.1553-2712.2008.00339.x

[33] Ely EW, Margolin R, Francis J, May L, Truman B, Dittus R, et al. Evaluation of delirium in critically ill patients: validation of the Confusion Assessment Method for the Intensive Care Unit (CAM-ICU). Crit Care Med. 2001 Jul;29(7):1370-9. DOI: 10.1097/00003246-200107000-00012

[34] Pfeiffer E. A short portable mental status questionnaire for the assessment of organic brain deficit in elderly patients. J Am Geriatr Soc. 1975 Oct;23(10):433-41. DOI: 10.1111/j.1532-5415.1975.tb00927.x

[35] Folstein MF, Folstein SE, McHugh PR. "Mini-mental state". A practical method for grading the cognitive state of patients for the clinician. J Psychiatr Res. 1975 Nov;12(3):189-98. doi: 10.1016/0022-3956(75)90026-6

[36] Nasreddine ZS, Phillips NA, Bedirian V, Charbonneau S, Whitehead V, Collin I, et al. The Montreal Cognitive Assessment, MoCA: a brief screening tool for mild cognitive impairment. J Am Geriatr Soc. 2005 Apr;53(4):695-9. DOI: 10.1111/j.1532-5415.2005.53221.x

[37] Borson S, Scanlan J, Brush M, Vitaliano P, Dokmak A. The mini-cog: a cognitive 'vital signs' measure for dementia screening in multi-lingual elderly. Int J Geriatr Psychiatry. 2000 Nov;15(11):1021-7. DOI: 10.1002/1099-1166(200011)15:11<1021::aid-gps234>3.0.co;2-6

[38] Witlox J, Eurelings LSM, de Jonghe JFM, Kalisvaart KJ, Eikelenboom P, van Gool WA. Delirium in Elderly Patients and the Risk of Postdischarge Mortality, Institutionalization, and Dementia: A Meta-analysis. JAMA. 2010;304(4):443-451. doi:10.1001/jama.2010.1013

[39] Rubin FH, Neal K, Fenlon K, Hassan S, Inouye SK. Sustainability and scalability of the hospital elder life program at a community hospital. J Am Geriatr Soc. 2011;59(2):359-365. doi:10.1111/j.1532-5415.2010.03243.x

[40] Wiffen P, Mitchell M, Snelling M, Stoner N, editors. Oxford Handbook of Clinical Pharmacy. 2. ed. New York: Oxford University Press, 2012. 674 p. DOI: 10.1093/med/9780199603640.001.0001

[41] Scott IA, Hilmer SN, Reeve E, Potter K, Le Couteur D, Rigby D, et al. Reducing inappropriate polypharmacy: The process of deprescribing. JAMA Internal Medicine. 2015; 175(5):827-834. DOI: 10.1001/jamainternmed.2015.0324

[42] Agbabiaka TB, Wider B, Watson LK, Goodman C. Concurrent Use of Prescription Drugs and Herbal Medicinal Products in Older Adults: A Systematic Review. Drugs and Aging. 2017; 34:891-905. DOI: 10.1007/s40266-017-0501-7

[43] Hshieh TT, Inouye SK, Oh ES. Delirium in the Elderly. Psychiatric Clinics of North America. 2018;41(1):1-17. DOI: 10.1016/j.psc.2017.10.001

[44] Sharma M, Loh KP, Nightingale G, Mohile SG, Holmes HM. Polypharmacy and potentially inappropriate medication use in geriatric oncology. Journal of Geriatric Oncology. 2016; 7(5):346-353. DOI: 10.1016/j.jgo.2016.07.010

[45] Morrison RS, Magaziner J, Gilbert M, Koval KJ, McLaughlin MA, Orosz G, Strauss E, Siu AL. Relationship between pain and opioid analgesics on the development of delirium following hip fracture. Journal of Gerontology: MEDICAL SCIENCES. 2003;58(1):76-81. DOI:10.1093/gerona/58.1.m76

[46] Alagiakrishnan K, Wiens CA. An approach to drug induced delirium in the elderly. Postgraduate Medical Journal. 2004;80:388-393. DOI: 10.1136/pgmj.2003.017236

[47] Fosnight S. Delirium in the elderly. In: Richardson MM, Chessman KH, Chant C., editors. Pharmacotherapy Self-Assessment Program. 7th ed. Lenexa: American College of Clinical Pharmacy; 2011. p. 73-96.

[48] AGS. American Geriatrics Society 2019 Updated AGS Beers Criteria® for Potentially Inappropriate Medication Use in Older Adults. Journal of the American Geriatrics Society. 2019;67(4):674-694. DOI: 10.1111/jgs.15767

[49] Salahudeen MS, Duffull SB, Nishtala PS. Anticholinergic burden quantified by anticholinergic risk scales and adverse outcomes in older people: A systematic review. BMC Geriatrics. 2015; 15:31. DOI: 10.1186/s12877-015-0029-9

[50] Catic AG. Identification and management of in-hospital drug-induced delirium in older patients. Drugs Aging. 2011;28(9):737-748. DOI:10.2165/11592240-000000000-00000

[51] Harrison PJ, Luciano S, Colbourne L. Rates of delirium associated with calcium channel blockers compared to diuretics, renin-angiotensin system agents and beta-blockers: An electronic health records network study. Journal of Psychopharmacology. 2020;34(8):848-855. DOI:10.1177/0269881120936501

[52] Zieschang T, Wolf M, Vellappallil T, Uhlmann L, Oster P, Kopf D. The Association of Hyponatremia, Risk of Confusional State, and Mortality. Dtsch Arztebl Int. 2016;113(50):855-862. DOI: 10.3238/arztebl.2016.0855

[53] Meyer S, Meyer O, Kressig RW. [Drug-induced delirium]. Therapeutische Umschau. Revue therapeutique. 2010;67(2):79-83. DOI: 10.1024/0040-5930/a000015

[54] Garpestad E, Devlin JW. Polypharmacy and Delirium in Critically Ill Older Adults: Recognition and Prevention. Clinics in Geriatric Medicine. 2017;33(2):189-203. DOI:10.1016/j.cger.2017.01.002

[55] Clegg A, Siddiqi N, Heaven A, Young J, Holt R. Interventions for preventing delirium in older people in institutional long-term care. Cochrane Database of Systematic Reviews. 2014; 1: CD009537. DOI: 10.1002/14651858.CD009537.pub2

[56] Kassie GM, Ellett LMK, Nguyen TA, Roughead EE. Current practice and opinions of hospital pharmacists regarding their role in the screening, prevention and treatment of delirium. International Journal of Clinical Pharmacy. 2017;39(6):1194-1200. DOI:10.1007/s11096-017-0547-y

[57] Motter FR, Fritzen JS, Hilmer SN, Paniz EV, Paniz VMV. Potentially inappropriate medication in the elderly: a systematic review of validated explicit criteria. European Journal of Clinical Pharmacology. 2018; 74: 679-700. DOI: 10.1007/s00228-018-2446-0

[58] O'Mahony D, O'Sullivan D, Byrne S, O'Connor MN, Ryan C, Gallagher P. STOPP/START criteria for potentially inappropriate prescribing in older people: Version 2. Age and Ageing. 2015; 44(2):213-218. DOI: 10.1093/ageing/afu145

[59] Nguyen PVQ, Pelletier L, Payot I, Latour J. Drug Delirium Scale (DDS): A tool to evaluate drugs as a risk fator for delirium. Internacional Journal of Innovative Reasearchin Medical Science. 2016;1(6):232-237. DOI:10.23958/ijirms/vol01-i06/02

[60] Nguyen PVQ, Pelletier L, Payot I, Latour J. The Delirium Drug Scale is associated to delirium incidence in the emergency department. International

Psychogeriatrics. 2018;30(4):503-510. DOI: 10.1017/S1041610217002538

[61] Nery RT, Reis AMM. Development of a Brazilian anticholinergic activity drug scale. einstein (São Paulo). 2019;17(2):eAO4435. DOI:10.31744/einstein_journal/2019AO4435

[62] Hwang S, Jun K, Ah YM, Han E, Chung JE, Lee JY. Impact of anticholinergic burden on emergency department visits among older adults in Korea: A national population cohort study. Archives of Gerontology and Geriatrics. 2019;85:103912. DOI: 10.1016/j.archger.2019.103912

[63] Machen S, Jani Y, Turner S, Marshall M, Fulop NJ. The role of organizational and professional cultures in medication safety: A scoping review of the literature. International Journal for Quality in Health Care. Oxford University Press; 2019. pp. G146–G157. DOI:10.1093/intqhc/mzz111

[64] Capucho HC, Carvalho FD, Cassiani SHDB. Farmacovigilância: Gerenciamento de Riscos da Terapia Medicamentosa para a Segurança do Paciente. 1st ed. São Caetano do Sul: Yendis; 2011

[65] Fong A, Harriott N, Walters DM, Foley H, Morrissey R, Ratwani RR. Integrating natural language processing expertise with patient safety event review committees to improve the analysis of medication events. Int J Med Inform. 2017;104: 120-125. DOI:10.1016/j.ijmedinf.2017.05.005

[66] Monteiro SAMG, Takano OA, Waldman EA. Evaluation of the Brazilian surveillance system for adverse events following vaccination. Rev Bras Epidemiol. 2011;14: 361-371. DOI:10.1590/S1415-790X2011000300002

[67] Sánchez A, Thomas C, Deeken F, Wagner S, Klöppel S, Kentischer F, et al. Patient safety, cost-effectiveness, and quality of life: reduction of delirium risk and postoperative cognitive dysfunction after elective procedures in older adults—study protocol for a stepped-wedge cluster randomized trial (PAWEL Study). Trials. 2019;20: 71. DOI:10.1186/s13063-018-3148-8

[68] Currow DC, Rowett D, Doogue M, To THM, Abernethy AP. An International Initiative To Create a Collaborative for Pharmacovigilance in Hospice and Palliative Care Clinical Practice. J Palliat Med. 2012;15: 282-286. DOI:10.1089/jpm.2012.9605

[69] Fornasier G, Francescon S, Leone R, Baldo P. An historical overview over Pharmacovigilance. Int J Clin Pharm. 2018;40: 744-747. DOI:10.1007/s11096-018-0657-1

Section 4

Scientific Methods and Tools for Safety Surveillance

Chapter 9

Computer-Aided Pharmacoepidemiology in Drug Use and Safety: Examining the Intersection between Data Science and Medicines Research

Ibrahim Chikowe and Elias Peter Mwakilama

Abstract

Pharmacoepidemiology is a relatively new area of study that focuses on research aimed at producing data about drugs' usage and safety in well-defined populations. Its significant impact on patient safety has translated into improving health care systems worldwide, where it has been widely adopted. This field has developed to an extent that policy and guidelines makers have started using its evidence alongside that produced from randomised controlled clinical trials. Although this significant improvement has been partly attributed to the adoption of statistics and computer-aided models into the way pharmacoepidemiology studies are designed and conducted, certain gaps still exist. This chapter reports some of the significant developments made, along with the gaps observed so far, in the adoption of statistics and computing into pharmacoepidemiology research. The goal is to highlight efforts that have led to the new pharmacoepidemiology developments, while examining the intersection between data science and pharmacology through research narrative reviews of computer-aided pharmacology. The chapter shows the significant number of initiatives that have been applied/adopted to improve pharmacoepidemiology research. Nonetheless, further developments in integrating pharmacoepidemiology with computers and statistics are needed in order to enhance the research agenda.

Keywords: Database, data science, computer-aided, pharmacovigilance, safety, adverse drug reaction

1. Introduction

Pharmacoepidemiology is a research field that applies epidemiological concepts into clinical pharmacology. It is important in the provision of an evidence base for pharmacotherapy, due to the abundance of digital data that is mostly scanty [1, 2]. Pharmacoepidemiology studies aim to quantify patterns of drug use, as well as adverse drug events, and include prescribing, use appropriateness, adherence to treatment regimen and persistence patterns, along with factors that assist in predicting medication use. In addition, pharmacoepidemiology studies involve drug

IntechOpen

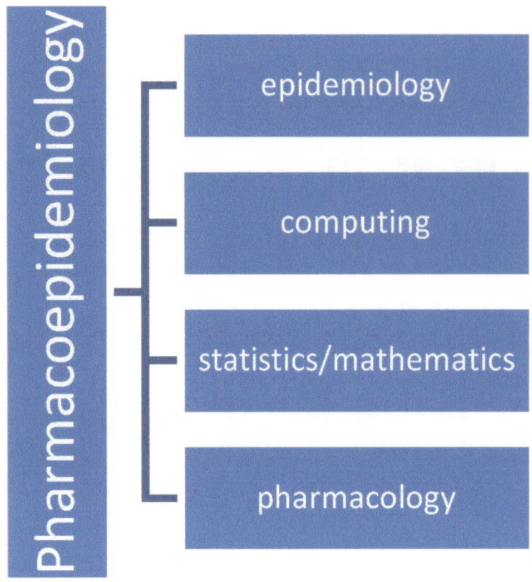

Figure 1.
Main contributors of Pharmacoepidemiology.

safety studies in large populations that focus on common and uncommon, as well as predictable and unpredictable, adverse drug reactions (ADRs) [3]. In this case, all the studies rely on meta-data sources, and include primary data, comprising national data sources and surveys or registries; and secondary data comprising administrative databases, claims databases, as well as primary care electronic health and medical records. **Figure 1** presents the general description of pharmacoepidemiology [4] being a multidisciplinary type of research field which intersects mathematical disciplines with pharmacology.

Recently, it has been established that clinical trial-oriented studies alone are mostly found to be insufficient to provide conclusive data about the drug's safety and occurrence of adverse effects in larger populations, especially the occurrence of idiosyncratic adverse events and other rare events. This is attributed to both the smaller populations and shorter time periods in which the medicines are tested. Additionally, the effectiveness of the medicines is not fully determined by the time the medicines are launched into the market. Post-marketing surveillance, with the help of either statistical or computing models on longitudinal data, becomes a critical tool for solving these challenges. Furthermore, it is important to highlight that adverse drug events and drug's efficacy can vary between clinical trial protocols and health care delivery systems [5–7]. Therefore, pharmacoepidemiology research data has found its way into many aspects of health care systems, such as policy making, drug utilisation and safety decision making, clinical trial design or validation, as well as guidance for the improvement of medical prescription by physicians. Additionally, it is also essential for research and project implementation, methodology development, vaccine and medical devices safety assessment, as well as for minimisation of medication errors and drug-induced toxicities [8].

2. Challenges and opportunities linked to pharmacoepidemiology

Pharmacoepidemiology research provides very important data for the benefit of patients' safety and care since the data generated is more informative and reliable when the study is well designed. Pharmacoepidemiology research offers many advantages, including the use of large patient samples and inclusion of subpopulations that are under research in uncontrolled conditions [1]. It also describes and estimates the risks and other drug safety or efficacy phenomena in practice [9]. Pharmacoepidemiology approaches make the studies cheaper and faster, when compared to the randomised controlled trials initially performed prior to marketing or after marketing, thus enabling the researchers to assess generic medications, as well as medications after a long period of use. The methods used in pharmacoepidemiology research can also be adapted for their use in pharmacovigilance to assist in unearthing unknown side effects or ADRs, together with the discovery of new drug usages [10].

However, pharmacoepidemiology research also has its own drawbacks, such as contamination of the data with confounding factors and many sources of bias (information bias, selection bias), due to the non-randomised nature of treatment selection, being harder to draw conclusions [1, 11]. In addition, although inclusion of statistical models into pharmacoepidemiology has been already seen, little is known about integrating pharmacology with community behaviour models, such as social networks. Nonetheless, different scholars have suggested several ways of improving pharmacoepidemiology research, including the use of active comparison groups and within-individual designs, as well as propensity scoring [12]. Additionally, pharmacoepidemiology studies have also been improved by triangulation of multiple analytical and data collection approaches, aiming to enhance the confidence in inferred causal relationships [13]. The developments made in the use of databases, computer and statistical models, and big data have led to enormous improvements in the robustness of pharmacoepidemiology studies and the production of reliable data that is being considered as good evidence for inclusion in guidelines, alongside data generated from randomised controlled trials [14].

Having shown that pharmacoepidemiology research is now producing data that is important for health care guidelines and policy development, it is essential that researchers can collaborate with guideline writers to ensure that they frame their questions to get useful answers. On the other hand, pharmacoepidemiology researchers should design their studies in such a way that guideline writers are provided with concrete answers, thus reducing the uncertainty in the evidence base. Additionally, since pharmacoepidemiology depends on statistical and data sciences, there is a need for further development of techniques in these fields to improve the application of pharmacoepidemiology. It is also important to enhance public engagement and capacity building (data resources and researcher base) to take full advantage of future opportunities [1].

3. Computational and statistical models in pharmacoepidemiology

The advent and development of computers has led to the development of databases that have become essential in pharmacoepidemiology. Several Electronic Health Records (EHRs) systems have been developed to keep longitudinal digital records of patient health information that are generated after a series of visits in a hospital setting [15]. EHRs contain patient data related to diseases, medicines and laboratory results, if any, and enable the provision of patient centred treatment by the health care providers [16, 17]. When these databases are linked or nationalised, it prevents patients repeatedly describing their medical histories, in case of treatment transfers. In addition, such data can be accessed by policy makers or researchers [18]. The use of computerised databases has led to a significant reduction in adverse events and prescription errors [19, 20], shorter hospital stays and lower mortality [21], along with better patient tracking, information exchange, efficient handling of information, and real-time data provision [16, 22]. Large pharmacoepidemiology data bases facilitate research, but they require well trained personnel to produce and handle big data [17, 23]. The use of electronic data has led to a significant reduction in the manual effort of data collection, easy incorporation of regional data into a study, minimal need for recalls, and removal of interviewer bias [24].

3.1 Progress and limitations

3.1.1 Usage of computational and statistical models

So far, a very close link between pharmacology and computational and statistical models has been established (**Figure 1**). In his work, Bentley [25] provides a well organised chapter describing the key statistical models used in the field of pharmacoepidemiology, both at descriptive and inferential analysis levels. Description uses measures of central tendency (e.g. mean), dispersion (e.g. variance), range (e.g. range, maximum and minimum), expressed in tables (e.g. cross-tabulations) and charts but inference may use regression models (e.g. linear, logistic, and Cox). These statistical techniques and descriptions aid in understanding data on usage and effects of drug administration at community level although it is also important to have a good knowledge of the potential errors involved in the design and analysis of pharmacoepidemiology studies [26].

Statistics play a major role in managing the quantifiable errors present in pharmacoepidemiology data analysis and interpretation [27]. Despite a growing interest in applying epidemiology statistical methods in pharmaceutical studies, a proper usage of the statistical techniques in research studies is often still lacking. For example, Suissa [26] states that pharmacoepidemiology observational research studies are hugely affected by information bias (when selecting variables of interest for the study), selection bias (during inclusion and exclusion of subjects), and confounding bias (due to imbalances in covariates). To circumvent these problems, both randomised controlled trials and cohort and case control studies, also used in epidemiological studies [28], have therefore been recommended by several researchers in pharmacoepidemiology [29].

Accordingly, in order to appraise the significance of epidemiological data and the design of studies on drug risk and safety, we reviewed a couple of research studies that have been conducted in developing countries, including in Malawi. We tried to focus on citing the key statistical and computational methods used in such research studies. To achieve this, we have used a similar approach to the one described by Sequi et al. [30] who presented a review of studies to underscore the processes of analysing and reporting data related to paediatric drug utilisation. Out of the 22 studies, the majority (91%) reported at least one descriptive measure, with the mean being the most common one (82%, 18/22), followed by the standard deviation (23%, 5/22). The chi-square test was observed in 12 studies, while graphical analysis was reported in 14 papers. However, only 16 papers reported the number of drug prescriptions and/or packages, while 10 reported the prevalence of the drug prescription. Consequently, the authors observed that only a few of the studies reviewed applied statistical methods and reported data in a satisfactory manner [27].

In a review paper which has set a position on current usage of statistical models in pharmacoepidemiology, Rosli and others [31] systematically reviewed published studies on drug utilisation in hospitalised neonates in Europe, the United States, India, Brazil, and Iran. The findings were not far from those reported by [30] such that a majority (70%) used descriptive statistics to analyse pharmacoepidemiology data. Nonetheless, some quite remarkable variations were observed regarding to the study design and methodology, sources of data, and sampling process among the selected studies. Of the included studies, 45% were based on cross-sectional or retrospective designs, 40% were prospective, and the remainder (15%) were point prevalence surveys.

Likewise, a 2020 review of 84 drug utilisation studies among neonates by Al-Turkait et al. [32] has shown that median, ranges and mean are frequently reported statistical parameters used for describing pharmacoepidemiology data, and that the style of reporting is mostly descriptive. However, in general public health, Hayat et al. [33] found a variety of statistical methods that were identified in the 216 papers reviewed, whereby 81.9% used an observational study design. 93.1% substantive analysis, 95% used descriptive statistics (tabular or graphical) while statistical inference (t-test, Chi-square, correlation with confidence intervals and p-values) was used in 76%. Logistic regression models were frequently used (38.4%), followed by linear regression models (19.4%).

Sequi et al. [30] recommended that the methodology of drug utilisation studies needs to be improved and we have also observed that drug use in the community is affected by drug availability, pricing, and affordability [34]. Therefore, the logistical and socio-economic aspects of pharmacoepidemiology studies should not be ignored. These two observations were the two key benchmarks for scoring the papers we have found and reviewed. For each study, we extracted information on the study design/type, data sources, period, assessment of variables used and corresponding statistical estimates (incidence, prevalence, pharmacy sales, prescription data), and diagnostic assessment. **Table 1** provides the overall summary details of the included papers.

By analysing **Table 1**, we have noticed that the status of pharmacoepidemiology research in some developing countries, like Malawi, is still at an infancy stage, compared to other developing countries that have adopted advanced inferential analyses into their pharmacoepidemiology research. Our findings do not differ from those reported by Sequi et al. [30], which the majority of the papers focused on the use of descriptive statistics. In addition, few studies clearly demonstrated the use of social/human behaviour network models in pharmacoepidemiology research [44, 45]. The inclusion of social/human behaviour network models into pharmacoepidemiology research is fundamental in the understanding of community structure and behaviour, for instance before mass drug administration during an outbreak such as COVID-19 [46, 47].

3.1.2 Big data in pharmacoepidemiology

Big data is another translational and frontier scientific discipline at the interface of computer science and statistics [48]. This field has found its way into pharmacoepidemiology research by simplifying the data interpretation and trend analysis of the volumes of data produced from many sources in health records [49]. With big data, pharmacoepidemiology research experts and data scientists detect ADRs, and collaborate in signal detection, verification and validation of medication or vaccine safety signals, as well as in the expansion of analytic methodologies for analysing the large volumes of heterogeneous data [14]. For example, the Exploring and Understanding Adverse Drug Reactions (EU-ADR) European project has incorporated innovative research methods in their pharmacovigilance research through the use of a web platform, aiming to provide advanced medication data exploration and assessment features. This enables data scientists and pharmacoepidemiology experts to mine EHRs for drug-events of their interest [4, 50].

Study type/design	Data source(s)	Year	Statistical methods	Variable(s) of interest	Reference
Cross-sectional	Survey questionnaire data	2018	Descriptive (percentages, frequencies, charts, median, ratios) *Excel*	Drug availability, Drug pricing, Affordability	[34]
Controlled trial	Articles	2017	-	Vaccination times, Dosage amounts	[35]
Cross-sectional	Prospective population census, passive surveillance, serological studies and healthcare utilisation surveys	2017	Descriptive (charts, percentages) *Stata*	Pathogen transmission, exposure and susceptibility	[36]
Randomisation	Basic survey	2019	Descriptive (percentages) *Excel & SPSS*	Drug abuse, Prevalence	[37]
Cohort	Anonymised patient record database	2013–2016	Descriptive (percentages), inferential-negative binomial regression (confidence intervals) *Stata*	Incidence and mortality ratios	[38]
Randomized Clinical Trial	Clinical data	2012	Descriptive (proportions), inferential (chi-square test, Kruskal-Wallis test, confidence intervals, incidence rate ratio, p-values, risk ratios) *Software- Stata*	Antiretroviral (ARV) usage, initiation	[39]
Key Informant Interviews (KII) and Focus Groups (FGs)	Recorded and transcribed qualitative data	2019	Thematic analysis *Software-NVivo*	Vaccination trials	[40]
Matched case–control study	Case–control study data	1993	Descriptive (tables, frequencies, percentages) and inferential (conditional logistic regression, relative risks, odds ratio, likelihood ratios, and confidence intervals) *Software- not mentioned*	BCG vaccine, efficacy, leprosy	[41]

DOI: http://dx.doi.org/10.5772/intechopen.98730

Study type/design	Data source(s)	Year	Statistical methods	Variable(s) of interest	Reference
Cross-sectional	Drug prescription data from hospital electronic database	2020	Descriptive (frequencies and percentages for categorical variables) and (means, medians, standard deviations (SD), and interquartile ranges (IQR) for continuous variables). Mean and SD were used for normal distribution and median and IQR were used for skewed distribution. *SPSS and Excel*	Drug utilization	[42]
Retrospective	Pharmacokinetic data of children > = 2 years and adults	2018	Both descriptive and inferential models (mean absolute error from non-linear statistical models) *Stata*	Drug dosing and clearance	[43]

Table 1.
A review of computer aided research studies and usage of statistical models in Pharmacoepidemiology.

3.2 Databases

3.2.1 Importance of databases

Apart from the statistical innovations that have been incorporated into pharmacoepidemiology research, computer databases, networks and software are also playing a critical role in enhancing the field of pharmacoepidemiology, and notable developments have been reported in North America, Europe, and the Asia-Pacific region [51]. The rapid development of computer-aided technology has led to the improvement of electronic health records, which have further led to the advancement of many databases that may be used locally or internationally. Consequently, this has allowed for the possibility of conducting pharmacoepidemiology studies using multiple databases in one or more countries [5]. Several mechanisms have been developed to ensure maximum benefit from the multinational databases and collaborations, such as the creation of research networks [5].

The use of multinational databases enables researchers and policy makers to compare how medications and medical devices are utilised and prescribed, as well as to compare their safety profiles in different settings [51]. It also allows the identification of the underlying factors for the differences or similarities observed, which may include different patient selection, delivery systems and genetic differences [51]. Moreover, it relates drug effects (beneficial or adverse) with differences in ethnic groups (receptor and cytochrome polymorphism effect) and lifestyle (such as dietary habits), among others [52].

Furthermore, the use of multiple databases has overcome sample size problems for rare exposures, outcomes of medications, or rare diseases [5]. While it is challenging to get sufficient power when studying one area, data from multiple databases increase the sample size, thus providing the required statistical power. Additionally, the general use of meta-data may help to solve problems experienced by some countries or areas that do not have their own policies, medications, or medical devices [53]. Therefore, multiple databases provide reference points for such cases. Multiple databases also provide a platform for collaboration and communication amongst researchers in different and distant nations, which has led to the advancement of research in pharmacoepidemiology [5].

3.2.2 Multi-database networks

According to Sturkenboom and Schink [51], electronic healthcare databases have allowed analyses of drug and vaccine utilisation, including investigations of comparative effectiveness and safety. Consequently, both local and international databases have been developed worldwide for use in pharmacoepidemiology. In North America, administrative databases, such as the Health Services Databases in Saskatchewan [54] and the Ontario Health Insurance Plan [55] in Canada, have been set up to manage health care delivery costs, with the fundamental purpose of allowing fiscal tracking and accounting for the delivery of health care from a payer perspective. In the USA, databases managed by Government payers for claims data, for instance Medicaid and Medicare, data are also used in research [56].

Since some of the databases do not cover the entire population, some research networks have been set-up to facilitate multi-database studies that can cover the whole nation. These include the Canadian Drug Safety and Effectiveness Network (CDSEN), set-up in 2007 by the Canadian government, which connects multiple researchers across Canada with expertise in pharmacoepidemiology research [57, 58] as well as the USA Food and Drug Administration (FDA), whom established a

Sentinel Initiative in 2008 with the purpose of refining safety signals that would enable the development of a scalable and transparent organisational structure to study the safety of medical products [59], mainly through the organisation of multiple databases managed via one research governance structure [5, 60].

Similar initiatives have also been adopted in Europe. The EU-ADR [61] was initiated by the European Commission to develop a drug safety surveillance system reliant on connections amongst databases in European countries. This initiative benefits from reliable clinical data obtained from the electronic healthcare records of over 30 million of patients within all the participating countries, thus ensuring an efficient analysis of drug safety issues. Another initiative adopted along the same lines is the Pharmacoepidemiology Research on Outcomes of Therapeutics by an European ConsorTium (PROTECT), which involves 19 collaborative international working groups, networks and research projects in Europe [62]. Nordic countries have established the Nordic Pharmaco-Epidemiological Network (NorPEN), aiming to promote research collaboration and initiate cross-country population-based comparative research in pharmacoepidemiology, for further promotion of safer medication use [63].

The Asian Pharmacoepidemiology Network (AsPEN) was formed in 2008 by four countries, namely Korea, Japan, Australia, and Taiwan, and has currently expanded to Singapore, China, India, Hong Kong, and Thailand [64]. The AsPEN [65] was created to provide mechanisms for supporting pharmacoepidemiology research in Asia, as well as to facilitate the identification and validation of emerging safety issues among the Asian countries. The diversity of the countries provides multi-cultural and ethnic sources of safety data [63, 64]. Nevertheless, this is still an ongoing process, as some countries are still developing their own databases and infrastructures. Special attention should be given to the challenges of handling such multi-complex meta-data, and may involve collaboration of mathematicians, statisticians, epidemiologists and computer scientists (**Figure 1**).

Research networks specialised in certain subpopulations have also been initiated with the goal of studying populations under-represented in clinical trials, such as children, older people, and pregnant women. The most notable networks established for this purpose comprise the Task-force in Europe for Drug Development for the Young (TEDDY) [66]; the European network of population-based registries for the surveillance of congenital anomalies (EUROCAT) [67], for providing early warnings of new teratogenic exposures on congenital anomalies; the Innovative Medicines Initiatives (IMI) [68], for fostering collaboration between different stakeholders (the European Union and the European pharmaceutical industry) in order to address growing challenges in bringing new medicines to market and the rapidly evolving healthcare landscape; the VACCINE.GRID [69], a global network of leading public health organisations concerned with vaccine benefits and risk assessment; and the International Society for Pharmacoepidemiology (ISPE), an international professional organisation dedicated to the open exchange of scientific information for the benefit of people, drug safety in pregnancy, vaccine safety and/or biologics safety [70].

Last but not least, we have also noticed that computational infrastructures have been developed in places where data participants can transform their data locally, as well as execute standardised analytical programs and combine the results [45]. Data science has also been exploited in pharmacoepidemiology research, where it is used in the evaluation of various analytical methods in the context of a network of databases [45, 47]. Common data models that are capable of accommodating heterogeneous databases and executing large-scale statistical analyses [71–73], whose resources sometimes can be downloaded from a website [74], have also been developed. **Table 2** illustrates a few databases that are currently being used as well

Database name	Host(s)	Design	Data	Location	Target population	Data coverage	Reference(s)
Electronic Patient Registration System	Queen Elizabeth Central Hospital	Multiple	Multiple	Malawi	Various	Vital signs data, treatment, demographic data, diagnostic information	[38]
IADB.nl		Multiple	Multiple	Netherlands	Over 500,000 people	Live and stillbirth pregnancy identification, medicine use data, prescriptions from 54 community pharmacies	[52]
DEFF Research Database	Ministry of science, Technology and innovation; Ministry of Culture; Ministry of Education	Multiple	Multiple	Denmark	Countrywide	Dispensed drugs, with potential for linkage to outcomes	[75]
Odense University Pharmacoepidemiological Database (OPED)	University of Southern Denmark	Multiple	Multiple	County of Funen in Denmark	Countrywide	Reimbursed prescriptions	[76]
Disease Analyser Patient Database		Multiple	Multiple	Germany	German, UK, French, and Austrian population	Diagnoses, prescriptions, risk factors (such as smoking and obesity), and laboratory values for approximately 10 million patients	[77]
German Longitudinal Prescription Database (LRx)		Multiple	Multiple	Germany	Countrywide	Diseases, drug utilisation, treatment costs, 60% of prescriptions reimbursed by statutory health insurance funds in Germany	[78]

DOI: http://dx.doi.org/10.5772/intechopen.98730

Database name	Host(s)	Design	Data	Location	Target population	Data coverage	Reference(s)
Database on Veterinary Clinical Research in Homeopathy.		Multiple	Multiple	Germany	Many	200 entries of randomised clinical trials, non-randomised clinical trials, observational studies, drug proving, case reports and case series	[79]
UK General Practice Research Database (GPRD).	UK Department of Health	Longitudinal	Case reports	UK	5 million patients; Countrywide	Collated information from over 500 general physicians' practices	[80, 81]
Clinical Research Database	Memorial Sloan-Kettering Cancer Center (MSKCC)	Multiple	Multiple		Patients on IRB approved studies who have passed through bone marrow transplant (BMT)	Diseases, pathology, infusion, treatment, among others.	[82]
Cancer Research DataBase (CRDB)	Cancer informatics project	Multiple	Mediation and data warehousing		Small molecule	Small molecule data, computational docking results, functional assays, and protein structure data	[83]
Danish Database for Biological Therapies in Rheumatology (DANBIO)	DANBIO	Multiple	Multiple	Denmark	Patients taking Biological treatments	Patients with rheumatoid arthritis (RA), psoriatic arthritis (PsA) and axial spondyloarthritis (Ax SpA), who are followed longitudinally	[84, 85]

Database name	Host(s)	Design	Data	Location	Target population	Data coverage	Reference(s)
The FoodCast Research Image Database (FRIDa)		Multiple	Multiple	Sweden	Wide range of foodstuff and related materials	877 images from eight different categories: natural-food, natural-non-food items. Artificial food-related objects	[86]
Pharmacy Dispensing Database		Multiple	Multiple	Netherlands, Denmark, Norway, Wales, France and Tuscany-Italy	Countrywide	Medicine use data	[87]
Danish National Patient Registry, Norway Medical Birth Registry		Multiple	Multiple	Norway and Denmark	Countrywide	Pregnancy loss identification	[87]
Influenza Research Database (IRD)	Bioinformatics Resource Center	Multiple	Multiple	US	All species of influenza virus sequence data	Influenza virus data, analytical and visualisation tools for influenza virus, personal workbenches for storing data	[88, 89]
Beth Israel Deaconess Medical Centre	Washington heart Centre, Beth Israel hospital, Boston	Multiple	Multiple	USA	Countrywide	Patient problems, medication, lab results	[90]
USDA's National Nutrient Database for Standard Reference, the Dietary Supplement Ingredient Database, the Food and Nutrient Database for Dietary Studies, and the USDA's Food Patterns Equivalents Database	US Department of Agriculture (USDA)	Multiple	Multiple	USA	Foodstuffs	Food and nutrients	[91]

Database name	Host(s)	Design	Data	Location	Target population	Data coverage	Reference(s)
Camden and Islington NHS Foundation Trust (C&I) Research Database	South London and Maussley NHS Foundation Trust (SLaM)	Multiple	Multiple	UK	Countrywide	108,168 mental health patients; 23,538 were receiving active care	[92]
Population and Housing Census (PHC), Health and Welfare Survey (HWS), Socio-Economic Survey (SES), Reproductive Health Survey (RHS), National Disability Survey (NDS), Multiple Indicator Cluster Survey (MICS)	National Statistics Office (NSO)	Interviews, face to face, self-enumeration, internet	Cross sectional	Thailand	Various	General population, health insurance, illness, health services, payment, equity, injury, co-morbidity, income, expenditure, debt, household distribution, family planning, maternal and child health. AIDS, Cancer, infertility, sex education, adolescent health	[93]
Cancer Registry	National Cancer Institute (NCI)	Longitudinal	Case reports	Thailand	All patients	Cancerous diseases, medicines	[93]
Thai Vigibase	Health Product Vigilance Centre (HPVC)		Case reports	Thailand	All patients	Adverse events	[93]
Adverse Events Database	Pharmaceutical and Medical Devices Agency (PMDA)		Case reports	Japan	Countrywide	Adverse events	[93]
National Community Pharmacy Group		Multiple	Multiple	South Africa	Countrywide	Drug utilisation	[94]

Database name	Host(s)	Design	Data	Location	Target population	Data coverage	Reference(s)
South African Medicine Claims Data	Pharmaceutical Benefit Management Company (PBM)	Multiple	Multiple	South Africa	Countrywide	Medicines claims	[95]
Strategic Typhoid Alliance Across Africa (STRATAA)				Malawi, Nepal, and Bangladesh	Countrywide	Demographic data, typhoid disease data	[96]
VigiBase	Uppsala Monitoring Centre (UMC)	Multiple	Multiple	Sweden	Worldwide	Adverse drug events	[97]
District Health Information System 2 (DHIS-2)	Kenya Medical Research Institute (KEMRI), Kamuzu Central Hospital	Multiple	Multiple	Kenya, Malawi, Uganda, Zambia [98]	Various	General health records and drug supply	[99, 100]
Mitishamba Database of Natural Products	University of Nairobi	Anti-Malaria drugs	Natural products	Kenya	Sub-Saharan Africa	Medicinal plants	[101]
International Databases to Evaluate AIDS (IeDEA-EA)	KEMRI, Mbarara Univ. & Tanzania	HIV-AIDS care	Drugs and Personal Protective Equipment (PPEs)	Kenya, Tanzania, Uganda	East African population	HIV care treatment	[102]

Table 2.
Computer databases currently used in pharmacoepidemiology research.

as those comprising data that may be potentially used to improve pharmacoepidemiology research. Although this is not an exhaustive list, these databases may serve as a supplement to those already reported [51].

Although the majority of pharmacoepidemiology research is found in developed countries, most of these databases are open for re-use of data, thus providing an opportunity for enhanced pharmacoepidemiology research, for instance in Asia and Africa [103].

3.2.3 Challenges with use of databases

Databases have limitations that affect their use in pharmacoepidemiology. Bias is one of the challenges and may be categorised into confounding, selection bias and time-related bias [98]. Confounding is further sub classified into confounding by indication, unmeasured or residual confounding, time-dependent confounding, and health user or adherer effect. Selection bias is reported to be associated with database use, being in the subcategories of protopathic bias, losses to follow up, prevalent user bias, and missing data. Another type of bias widely reported is measurement bias, which comes in the form of miscalculation bias, miscalculation of exposure, as well as miscalculation of outcomes. Time-related bias is classified into immortal bias, immeasurable time bias, time-window bias and time-lag bias [98].

4. Conclusions

Through a cross-examination of the intersection between data science principles and pharmacoepidemiology, this chapter has demonstrated that pharmacoepidemiology has greatly evolved over the years, from being a mere research field to one that is playing a significant role in the enhancement of patient safety, as well as in the development of health care guidelines and policies. Our examination of the intersection between data science techniques and pharmacoepidemiology was limited to the policy and research narratives of computer-aided pharmacoepidemiology studies across the globe. The level of evidence generated from several studies indicates that the field is now as important as randomised clinical trials have been, which can be attributed to the adoption of statistical and computational principles and practices. However, it is important to highlight that, although there has been a significant number of initiatives reported to improve pharmacoepidemiology research, the identified gaps and challenges presented in this chapter show that this field still has some potential to grow, for instance by properly integrating the existing data science techniques with appropriate principles and practices. The inclusion of both logistical and social/human behaviour network models into pharmacoepidemiology is strongly recommended.

Acknowledgements

This publication was made possible with funding from the Agency for Scientific Research and Training (ASRT) in Malawi. Sincere thanks are due to Dr. David Scott for the technical, language editing and proofreading support on the manuscript.

Author contributions

IC conceived the study, performed the review of pharmacoepidemiology databases and participated in the manuscript writing process. EM reshaped the argument of the study, reviewed research papers on statistical and computing models, and participated in the manuscript writing process. All authors have read and approved the final manuscript.

Conflict of interest

The authors declare no conflict of interest.

Appendices and nomenclature

ADRs	Adverse Drug Reactions
AIDS	Acquired Immunodeficiency Syndrome
ARV	Antiretroviral drugs
AsPEN	Asian Pharmacoepidemiology Network
BCG	BCG-Bacille Calmette-Guerin
BMT	Bone Marrow Transplant
CDSEN	Canadian Drug Safety and Effectiveness Network
COVID-19	Coronavirus Disease 2019
DANBIO	Danish Database for Biological Therapies in Rheumatology
DHIS-2	District Health Information System (version 2)
EHRs	Electronic Health Records
EU-ADR	Exploring and Understanding Adverse Drug Reactions
EUROCAT	European Network of Population-based Registries for the Surveillance of Congenital Anomalies
FDA	Food and Drug Administration
FGD	Focus Groups Discussion
FRIDa	The FoodCast Research Image Database
GPRD	UK General Practice Research Database
HPVC	Health Product Vigilance Centre
HWS	Health and Welfare Survey
IADB.nl	InterAction Database
IeDEA-EA	East African International Databases to Evaluate AIDS
IMI	Innovative Medicines Initiatives
IQR	Interquartile Range
IRD	Influenza Research Database
ISPE	International Society for Pharmacoepidemiology
KIIs	Key Informant Interviews
MICS	Multiple Indicator Cluster Survey
MSKCC	Memorial Sloan-Kettering Cancer Centre
NCI	National Cancer Institute
NDS	National Disability Survey
NorPEN	Nordic Pharmaco- Epidemiological Network
NSO	National Statistical Office
OPED	Odense University Pharmacoepidemiological Database
PBM	Pharmaceutical Benefit Management Company
PHC	Population and Housing Census
PMDA	Pharmaceutical and Medical Devices Agency
PROTECT	Research on Outcomes of Therapeutics by an European ConsorTium
RHS	Reproductive Health Survey
SD	Standard Deviations

SES	Socio-Economic Survey
SPSS	Statistical Package for Social Scientists
STRATAA	Strategic Typhoid Alliance across Africa
TEDDY	Task-force in Europe for Drug Development for the Young
USDA	U.S. Department of Agriculture

Author details

Ibrahim Chikowe[1]* and Elias Peter Mwakilama[2]

1 Pharmacy Department, College of Medicine, University of Malawi, Blantyre, Malawi

2 Mathematical Sciences Department, Chancellor College, University of Malawi, Zomba, Malawi

*Address all correspondence to: chikoweib@yahoo.co.uk; ichikowe@medcol.mw

References

[1] Davis KAS, Farooq S, Hayes JF, John A, Lee W, MacCabe JH, et al. Pharmacoepidemiology research: delivering evidence about drug safety and effectiveness in mental health. The Lancet Psychiatry. 2020;7(4):363-370.

[2] Salas M, Stricker B. Research Methods for Pharmacoepidemiology Studies. In: S.P. G, editor. Essentials of Clinical Research [Internet]. Dordrecht: Springer; 2008. p. 201-16. Available from: https://doi.org/10.1007/978-1-4020-8486-7_12

[3] Yang Y, West-Strum D. Introduction to Pharmacoepidemiology. In: Yang Y, West-Strum D, editors. Understanding Pharmacoepidemiology. 1st ed. McGraw Hill; 2011.

[4] Nishtala P. Sources of data used in pharmacoepidemiology and pharmacovigilance. Elsevier [Internet]. 2019;391. Available from: https://doi.org/10.1016/B978-0-12-812735-3.00206-5

[5] Lai EC-C, Stang P, Yang Y-HK, Kubota K, Wong ICK, Setoguchi S. International Multi-database Pharmacoepidemiology: Potentials and Pitfalls. Curr Epidemiol Reports. 2015;2(4):229-38.

[6] Lasser KE, Allen PD, Woolhandler SJ, Himmelstein DU, Wolfe SM, Bor DH. Timing of new black box warnings and withdrawals for prescription medications. J Am Med Assoc. 2002; 287(17):2215-20.

[7] Strom BL, Carson JL. Use of Automated Databases for Pharmacoepidemiology Research. Epidemiol Rev [Internet]. 1990 Jan 1;12(1):87-107. Available from: https://doi.org/10.1093/oxfordjournals.epirev.a036064

[8] Lee D, Majumdar SR, Levens H, B. LS, Sean S, L. HR, et al. Special applications of pharmacoepidemiology. In: Strom BL, Kimmel SE, editors. Textbook of Pharmacoepidemio logy. 2006.

[9] Nour S, Plourde G. Pharmaco epidemiology in the prevention of adverse drug reactions. In: Nour S, Plourde G, editors. Pharmaco epidemiology and pharmacovigilance [Internet]. Elsevier Inc.; 2019. p. 25-65. Available from: https://doi.org/10.1016/C2017-0-04746-8

[10] Faillie JL, Montastruc F, Montastruc JL, Pariente A. Pharmaco epidemiology and its input to pharmacovigilance. Therapie [Internet]. 2016;71(2):211-216,. Available from: https://doi.org/10.1016/j.therap.2016.02.016

[11] Wettermark B. The intriguing future of pharmacoepidemiology. Eur J Clin Pharmacol [Internet]. 2013;69:43-51,. Available from: https://doi.org/10.1007/s00228-013-1496-6

[12] Suissa S. Statistical Methods in Pharmacoepidemiology. Drug-Safety [Internet]. 1991;6:381-389. Available from: https://doi.org/10.2165/00002018-199106050-00008

[13] Hopf YM, Francis J, Helms PJ, Haughney J, Bond C. Core requirements for successful data linkage: An example of a triangulation method. BMJ Open. 2016;6(10).

[14] Sánchez-Duque JA, Gaviria-Mendoza A, Moreno-Gutiérrez PA, Machado-Alba JE. Big data, pharmacoepidemiology and pharmacovigilance. Rev Fac Med. 2020;68(1):117-20.

[15] Masnoon N, Shakib S, Kalisch-Ellett L, Al. E. Tools for Assessment of the Appropriateness of Prescribing and Association with Patient-Related

Outcomes: A Systematic Review. Drugs Aging [Internet]. 2018;35:43-60. Available from: https://doi.org/10.1007/s40266-018-0516-8

[16] Deloitte. Independent review of New Zealand's Electronic Health Records Strategy [Internet]. New Zealand: Deloite; 2015. Available from: https://www.health.govt.nz/system/files/documents/publications/independent-review-new-zealand-electronic-health-records-strategy-oct15.pdf

[17] Murray MD. Use of Data from Electronic Health Records for Pharmacoepidemiology. Curr Epidemiol Reports. 2014;1(4):186-93.

[18] MOH. Electronic Health Record [Internet]. 2021 [cited 2021 Mar 20]. Available from: https://www.health.govt.nz/our-work/ehealth/digital-health-2020/electronic-health-record

[19] Charles K, Cannon M, Hall R, Coustasse A. Can utilizing a computerized provider order entry (CPOE) system prevent hospital medical errors and adverse drug events? Perspect Health Inf Manag. 2014;11(March 2012).

[20] Nuckols TK, Smith-Spangler C, Morton SC, Asch SM, Patel VM, Anderson LJ, et al. The effectiveness of computerized order entry at reducing preventable adverse drug events and medication errors in hospital settings: A systematic review and meta-analysis. Syst Rev. 2014;3(1):1-12.

[21] Prgomet M, Li L, Niazkhani Z, Georgiou A, Westbrook JI. Impact of commercial computerized provider order entry (CPOE) and clinical decision support systems (CDSSs) on medication errors, length of stay, and mortality in intensive care units: A systematic review and meta-analysis. J Am Med Informatics Assoc. 2017;24(2):413-22.

[22] Harpe SE. Using secondary data sources for pharmacoepidemiology and outcomes research. Pharmacotherapy. 2009;29(2):138-53.

[23] Torre C, Martins AP. Overview of pharmacoepidemiological databases in the assessment of medicines under real-life conditions. In: Lunet N, editor. Current Perspectives on Research and Practice. IntechOpen; 2012. p. 186-193,.

[24] Sink KM, Thomas J, Xu H, Craig B, Kritchevsky S, Sands LP. Dual Use of Bladder Anticholinergics and Cholinesterase Inhibitors: Long-Term Functional and Cognitive Outcomes Kaycee. J Am Geriatr Soc. 2015;33(4): 395-401.

[25] Bentley JP. Biostatistics and Pharmacoepidemiology. In: Yang Y, West-Strum D, editors. Understanding Pharmacoepidemiology. New York: McGraw-Hill; 2011. p. 79-104.

[26] Suissa S. Statistical methods in pharmacoepidemiology: Advances and challenges. Stat Methods Med Res. 2009;18(1):3-6.

[27] Liu R, Tsong Y. Pharmaceutical Statistics. 1st ed. Vol. 218, MBSW 39, Muncie, Indiana, USA, May 16-18, 2016. Muncie, Indiana, USA: Springer International Publishing; 2019. XI, 337.

[28] Filardo G, Adams J, Keung HNT. Statistical Methods in Epidemiology. In: M. L, editor. International Encyclopedia of Statistical Science. Berlin, Heidelberg: Springer; 2011.

[29] Replicable WD, Non R, Wang S, Rassen J, Pinheiro S, Berlin J, et al. Abstracts of the 35th International Conference on Pharmacoepidemiology & Therapeutic Risk Management, Pennsylvania Convention Center, Philadelphia, PA, USA, August 24-28, 2019. Pharmacoepidemiol Drug Saf. 2019;28:5-586.

[30] Sequi M, Campi R, Clavenna A, Bonati M. Methods in pharmaco epidemiology: A review of statistical analyses and data reporting in pediatric drug utilization studies. Eur J Clin Pharmacol. 2013;69(3):599-604.

[31] Rosli R, Dali AF, Aziz NA, Abdullah AH, Ming LC, Manan MM. Drug utilization on neonatal wards: A systematic review of observational studies. Front Pharmacol. 2017;8(FEB).

[32] Al-Turkait A, Szatkowski L, Choonara I, Ojha S. Review of Drug Utilization Studies in Neonatal Units: A Global Perspective. Int J Environ Res Public Health. 2020;17(16):56-69.

[33] Hayat MJ, Powell A, Johnson T, Cadwell BL. Statistical methods used in the public health literature and implications for training of public health professionals. PLoS One. 2020;12(6).

[34] Khuluza F, Haefele-Abah C. The availability, prices and affordability of essential medicines in Malawi: A cross-sectional study. PLoS One. 2019;14(2):1-22.

[35] Gordon SB, Rylance J, Luck A, Jambo K, Ferreira DM, Manda-Taylor L, et al. A framework for Controlled Human Infection Model (CHIM) studies in Malawi: Report of a Wellcome Trust workshop on CHIM in Low Income Countries held in Blantyre, Malawi. Wellcome Open Res. 2017;2(0):1-11.

[36] Darton TC, Meiring JE, Tonks S, Khan MA, Khanam F, Shakya M, et al. The STRATAA study protocol: A programme to assess the burden of enteric fever in Bangladesh, Malawi and Nepal using prospective population census, passive surveillance, serological studies and healthcare utilisation surveys. BMJ Open. 2017;7(6):1-9.

[37] Kuyokwa J, Chiziwa S, Chinkhata M, Muyila D. Epidemiology of Psychoactive Substance Use and Associated Factors among Adolescents: A Descriptive Study of Selected Secondary Schools in South West Education Division, Blantyre, Malawi. Integr J Glob Heal. 2019;3(1:1).

[38] Lewis JM, Abouyannis M, Katha G, Nyirenda M, Chatsika G, Feasey NA, et al. Population Incidence and Mortality of Sepsis in an Urban African Setting, 2013-2016. Clin Infect Dis. 2020;10(1):2547-2552,.

[39] MacPherson P, Lalloo DG, Webb EL, Maheswaran H, Choko AT, Makombe SD, et al. Effect of optional home initiation of HIV care following HIV self-testing on antiretroviral therapy initiation among adults in Malawi: A randomized clinical trial. JAMA - J Am Med Assoc. 2014;312(4): 372-9.

[40] Kapumba BM, Jambo K, Rylance J, Gmeiner M, Sambakunsi R, Parker M, et al. Stakeholder views on the acceptability of human infection studies in Malawi. BMC Med Ethics. 2020;21(1):1-15.

[41] Baker DM, Nguyen-Van-Tam JS, Smith SJ. Protective efficacy of BCG vaccine against leprosy in southern Malaŵi. Epidemiol Infect. 1993;111(1): 21-5.

[42] Yue Y, Chen L, Choonara I, Xiong T, Ojha S, Tang J, et al. Cross-sectional study of drug utilisation in a Chinese neonatal unit. J Int Med Res [Internet]. 2020;48(5):1-15. Available from: https://doi.org/10.1177/0300060520914197

[43] Tegenge MA, Mahmood I, Jiang Z, Forshee R. Multistep Unified Models Using Prior Knowledge for the Prediction of Drug Clearance in Neonates and Infants. J Clin Pharmacol. 2018;58(7):877-884.

[44] Kiss IZ, Miller J, Simon PL. Mathematics of Epidemics on Networks:

From Exact to Approximate Models. 1st ed. Switzerland: Springer International Publishing; 2017. 413,.

[45] Broeck W V.D., Gioannini C, Gonçalves B, Quaggiotto M, Colizza V, Vespignani A. The GLEaMviz computational tool, a publicly available software to explore realistic epidemic spreading scenarios at the global scale. BMC Infect Dis. 2011;11.

[46] Li MY. An Introduction to Mathematical Modeling of Infectious Diseases. 1st ed. Vol. 2, Mathematics of Planet Earth. Switzerland: Springer International Publishing; 2018. 156.

[47] Xu B, Kraemer MUG, Gutierrez B, Mekaru S, Sewalk K, Loskill A, et al. Open access epidemiological data from the COVID-19 outbreak. Lancet Infect Dis. 2020;20(5):534.

[48] Mayer-Schönberger V, Cukier K. Big Data: A Revolution That Will Transform How We Live, Work, and Think. Reprint. New York: Eamon Dolan/Mariner Books. ISBN-10; 2014. 544227751 p.

[49] Piontti AP y, Perra N, Rossi L, Samay N, Vespignani A. Charting the Next Pandemic: Modeling Infectious Disease Spreading in the Data Science Age. 1st ed. Switzerland: Springer International Publishing; 2019. 209,.

[50] Oliveira JL, Lopes P, Nunes T, Campos D, Boyer S, Ahlberg E, et al. The EU-ADR Web Platform: delivering advanced pharmacovigilance tools. Pharmacoepidemiol Drug Saf. 2013;22:459-467,.

[51] Sturkenboom M, Schink T. Databases for Pharmacoepidemiological Research. 1st ed. Switzerland: Springer International Publishing; 2021. 280 p.

[52] Visser ST, Schuiling-Veninga CC, Bos JH, Postma MJ, Berg LT de J den. The population-based prescription database IADB.nl: its development, usefulness in outcomes research and challenges. Expert Rev Pharmacoecon Outcomes Res. 2013;13(3):285-292,.

[53] Hennessy S. Use of Health Care Databases in Pharmacoepidemiology. Basic Clin Pharmacol Toxicol. 2006;98:311-313.

[54] Zuiderwijk A, Jeffery K, Janssen M. The Potential of Metadata for Linked Open Data and its Value for Users and Publishers. J e-Democracy Open Gov. 2012;4(2):222-244 ,.

[55] Fry RB, Ray MN, Cobaugh DJ, Weissman NW, Kiefe CI, Shewchuk RM, et al. Racial/ethnic disparities in patient-reported nonsteroidal antiinflammatory drug (NSAID) risk awareness, patient-doctor NSAID risk communication, and NSAID risk behavior. Arthritis Care Res. 2007;57(8):1539-45.

[56] Scales DC, Guan J, Martin CM, Redelmeier DA. Administrative data accurately identified intensive care unit admissions in Ontario. J Clin Epidemiol. 2006;59(8):802-7,.

[57] Hippisley-Cox J. Predicting risk of upper gastrointestinal bleed and intracranial bleed with anticoagulants: Cohort study to derive and validate the QBleed scores. BMJ [Internet]. 2014;349(July):1-21. Available from: http://dx.doi.org/doi:10.1136/bmj.g4606

[58] Lexchin J, Wiktorowicz M, Moscou K, Eggertson L. Provincial drug plan officials' views of the Canadian drug safety system. J Heal Polit Policy Law. 2013;38(3):545-71,.

[59] De Mello NR, Baracat EC, Tomaz G, Bedone AJ, Camargos A, Barbosa IC, et al. Double-blind study to evaluate efficacy and safety of meloxicam 7.5 mg and 15 mg versus mefenamic acid 1500 mg in the treatment of primary dysmenorrhea. Acta Obstet Gynecol Scand. 2004;83(7):667-73.

[60] Platt R, Carnahan RM, Brown JS, Chrischilles E, Curtis LH, Hennessy S, et al. The U.S. Food and Drug Administration's Mini-Sentinel program: status and direction. Pharmacoepidemiol Drug Saf. 2012;21(Suppl 1):1-8.

[61] EU-ADR. Exploring and Understanding Adverse Drug Reactions by Integrative Mining of Clinical Records and Biomedical Knowledge [Internet]. Exploring and Understanding Adverse Drug Reactions. 2020. Available from: http://www.euadr-project.org

[62] Sabaté M, Pacheco JF, Ballarín E, Ferrer P, Petri H, Hasford J, et al. A compilation of research working groups on drug utilisation across Europe. BMC Res Notes. 2014;7(1):1-5.

[63] Furu K, Wettermark B, Andersen M, Martikainen JE, Almarsdottir AB, Sørensen HT. The Nordic Countries as a Cohort for Pharmacoepidemiological Research. Basic Clin Pharmacol Toxicol. 2010;106(2):86-94.

[64] Andersen M, Bergman U, Choi N-K, Gerhard T, Huang C, Jalbert J, et al. The Asian Pharmacoepidemiology Network (AsPEN): promoting multi-national collaboration for pharmaco epidemiologic research in Asia. Pharmacoepidemiol Drug Saf. 2013;22(7):700-4,.

[65] AsPEN. Asian Pharmaco epidemiology Network [Internet]. Databases in Asia: The Potential for Distributed Network Approach. 2018 [cited 2021 May 16]. Available from: https://aspennet.asia/

[66] Ceci A, Giaquinto C, Aboulker J-P, Baiardi P, Bonifazi F, Pasqua O Della, et al. The Task-force in Europe for Drug Development for the Young (TEDDY) Network of Excellence. Pediatr Drugs Vol [Internet]. 2009;11:18-21. Available from: https://doi.org/10.2165/0148581-200911010-00008

[67] Dolk H. EUROCAT: 25 Years of European surveillance of congenital anomalies. Arch Dis Child Fetal Neonatal Ed. 2005;90(5):355-8.

[68] Laverty H, Meulien P. The Innovative Medicines Initiative –10 Years of Public-Private Collaboration. Front Med. 2019;6(December):1-13.

[69] Grid. V. No Title [Internet]. [cited 2021 May 16]. Available from: http://www.vaccinegrid.org/public.html.

[70] ISPE. International Society for Pharmacoepidemiology [Internet]. [cited 2021 May 16]. Available from: https://www.pharmacoepi.org/

[71] Paris N, Parrot A. MIMIC in the OMOP Common Data Model. medRxiv [Internet]. 2020;(Cdm):2020.08.14.20175141. Available from: https://doi.org/10.1101/2020.08.14.20175141

[72] Matcho A, Ryan P, Fife D, Reich C. Fidelity assessment of a clinical practice research datalink conversion to the OMOP Common Data Model. Drug Saf Int J Med Toxicol Drug Exp. 2014;37(11):945-59 ,.

[73] Makadia R, Ryan PB. Transforming the premier perspective hospital database into the Observational Medical Outcomes Partnership (OMOP) Common Data Model. EGEMS (Wash DC). 2010;2(1):1110.

[74] Overhage JM, Ryan PB, Reich CG, Hartzema AG, Stang PE. Validation of a common data model for active safety surveillance research. J Am Med Inf Assoc. 2012;19(1):54-60,.

[75] Wettermark B, Zoëga H, Furu K, Korhonen M, Hallas J, Nørgaard M, et al. The nordic prescription databases as a resurce for pharmacoepidemiological research-a literature review.

Pharmacoepidemiol Drug Saf. 2013;22(7):691-699,.

[76] Hallas J, Hellfritzsch M, Rix M, Olesen M, Reilev M, Pottegård A. Osense pharmacoepidemiological database: A review of use and content. Basic Clin Pharmacol Toxicol. 2017;120(5):419-425,.

[77] Becher H, Kostev K, Schröder-Bernhardi D. Validity and representativeness of the Disease Analyser patient database for use in pharmacoepidemiological and pharmacoeconomic studies. Int J Clin Pharmacol Ther. 2009;47(10): 617-626,.

[78] Richter H, Dombrowski S, Hamer H, Hadji P, Kostev K. Use of a German longitudinal prescription database (LRx) in pharmaco epidemiology. Ger Med Sci. 2015;13 (Doc14).

[79] Clausen J, Albrecht H. Database on veterinary clinical research in homeopathy. Homeopathy. 2010;99(3):189-191,.

[80] Bradley SH, Lawrence NR, Carder P. Using primary care data for health research in England – an overview. Futur Healthc J. 2018;5(3):207-12.

[81] Chen YC, Wu JC, Haschler I, Majeed A, Chen TJ, Wetter T. Academic impact of a public electronic health database: Bibliometric analysis of studies using the general practice research database. PLoS One. 2011;6(6):1-7.

[82] Latif M, Maloy M, Klein E, Fuller K, Truong H, Krishtul R. Redesign of an in house electronic data capture system to streamline hematopoietic stem cell informatics needs: Safeguarding over 40 years of data. Biol blood marrow Transplant [Internet]. 2019;25(3):269. Available from: https://doi.org/10.1016/j.bbmt.2018.12.210

[83] Bichutskiy VY, Colman R, Brachmann RK, Lathrop RH. Heterogeneous biomedical database integration using a hybrid strategy: A p53 cancer research database. Cancer Inform. 2006;2(949):277-87.

[84] Hetland ML. DANBIO-powerful research database and electronic patient record. Rheumatol. 2011;50(1):69-77,.

[85] Ibfelt EH, Jensen DV, Hetland ML. The Danish nationwide clinical register for patients with rheumatoid arthritis: DANBIO. Clin Epidemiol. 2016;8: 737-742,.

[86] Foroni F, Pergola G, Argiris G, Rumiati RI. The foodcast research image database (FRIDa). Front Hum Neurosci. 2013;7(FEB):1-19.

[87] Charlton RA, Neville AJ, Jordan S, Pierini A, Damase-Michel C, Klungsøyr K, et al. Healthcare databases in Europe for studying medicine use and safety during pregnancy. Pharmacoepidemiol Drug Saf. 2014;23:586-594.

[88] Rigden DJ, Fernández XM. The 27th annual Nucleic Acids Research database issue and molecular biology database collection. Nucleic Acids Res. 2020;48(D1):D1-8.

[89] Rigden DJ, Fernández XM. The 2018 Nucleic Acids Research database issue and the online molecular biology database collection. Nucleic Acids Res. 2018;46(D1):D1-7.

[90] Halamka JD. Early experiences with big data at an academic medical center. Health Aff. 2014;33(7):1132-8.

[91] Ahuja JKC, Moshfegh AJ, Holden JM, Harris E. USDA food and nutrient databases provide the infrastructure for food and nutrition research, policy, and practice. J Nutr. 2013;143(2):241-9.

[92] Werbeloff N, Osborn DPJ, Patel R, Taylor M, Stewart R, Broadbent M, et al. The camden & Islington research database: Using electronic mental health records for research. PLoS One. 2018;13(1):1-13.

[93] Saokaew S, Sugimoto T, Kamae I, Pratoomsoot C, Chaiyakunapruk N. Healthcare databases in Thailand and Japan: Potential sources for health technology assessment research. PLoS One [Internet]. 2015;10(11):1-20. Available from: http://dx.doi.org/10.1371/journal.pone.0141993

[94] Truter I. Antimicrobial prescribing in Southafrica using a large pharmacy database: A drug utilisation study IIse Truter. J Infect Dis [Internet]. 2014;30(2):52-56,. Available from: https://doi.org/10.1080/23120053.2015.1054181

[95] Obeng-Kusi M. Research methods for conducting pharmaco epidemiological studies using medicines claims data [Internet]. Masters Degree Dissertation. Northwest University; 2019. Available from: http://hdl.handle.net/10394/32816

[96] Thindwa D, Farooq YG, Shakya M, Saha N, Tonks S, Anokwa Y. Electronic data capture for large scale typhoid surveillance, household contact tracing, and health utilisation survey : strategic typhoid alliance across africa and asia. Wellcome Open Res. 2020;5(66).

[97] Ampadu HH, Hoekman J, de Bruin ML, Pal SN, Olsson S, Sartori D, et al. Adverse Drug Reaction Reporting in Africa and a Comparison of Individual Case Safety Report Characteristics Between Africa and the Rest of the World: Analyses of Spontaneous Reports in VigiBase®. Drug Saf. 2016;39(4):335-45.

[98] Prada-Ramallal G, Takkouche B, Figueiras A. Bias in pharmaco epidemiologic studies using secondary health care databases: a scoping review. BMC Med Res Methodol [Internet]. 2019;19(53). Available from: https://doi.org/10.1186/s12874-019-0695-y

[99] Chikumba P. Management of Health Information in Malawi: Role of Technology. Adv Sci Technol Eng Syst J. 2017;2:157-166 ,.

[100] Aywak D, Jaguga CDP, Nkonge NG, Kinuthia R, Ambale C, Awle IA. Pharmacy Practice in Kenya. Can J Hosp Pharm. 2017;70(6): 456-462 ,.

[101] Noor AM, Alegana VA, Gething PW, Snow RW. A spatial national health facility database for public health sector planning in Kenya in 2008. Int J Heal Geogr. 2009;8(13).

[102] ISPM. International Databases to Evaluate AIDS (IeDEA-EA) [Internet]. 2021 [cited 2021 Mar 17]. Available from: https://www.iedea.org/regions/east-africa/

[103] Alarkawi D, Ali MS, Bliuc D, Center JR, Prieto-Alhambra D. The Challenges and Opportunities of Pharmacoepidemiology in Bone Diseases. JBMR Plus. 2018;2(4):187-94.

Chapter 10

Basics and Essentials of Medical Devices Safety Surveillance

Vivekanandan Kalaiselven, Shatrunajay Shukla, Nikita Mishra and Pawan Kumar

Abstract

Medical devices are being used in healthcare facilities for diagnosis, monitoring, prevention and treatment of an array of diseases. To ensure user/patient safety associated with the medical devices being used in healthcare industry, it is of utmost importance to closely monitor the adverse events associated with the medical devices through a robust, sustainable and scaled surveillance. Materiovigilance Programme of India (MvPI) provides a reliable system to report adverse events associated with medical devices. Under MvPI, various modalities to report adverse events associated with medical devices have been developed. These modalities include an editable medical device adverse event reporting form, a toll-free helpline number and a field safety corrective action form (FSCA). FSCA form is used to notify the regulatory authority and healthcare professionals on corrective actions or recall by the manufacturer. Due to the emergence of the Coronavirus disease 2019 (COVID-19) pandemic, one-page editable form has been developed to boost the adverse event reporting of Personal Protective Equipments (PPEs). MvPI also coordinates with healthcare facilities and medical device industries across the country for reporting the medical device-related adverse events. The collected scientific data is utilized to develop regulatory policies and enhance measures to ensure the quality of medical devices. All the healthcare workers are, therefore, encouraged to report adverse events to MvPI. This chapter aims to describe the systems, procedures and modalities available for the reporting of Medical Device Adverse Events (MDAEs) in India, in order to intensify the nature of reporting and creating an environment that encourages the public to perform MDAE reporting.

Keywords: Adverse event, COVID-19, Materiovigilance Programme of India, Personal Protective Equipments, Causality assessment, Medical device

1. Introduction

Over the last years, medical devices have been playing a pivotal role in the diagnosis and management of a variety of diseases [1]. With the advancement in the technology and increased public demand for high quality medical care, the global medical device industry has surpassed USD 350 billion in annual revenue, and in India a growth rate of 20% has been seen in healthcare industry. These devices have also created substantial risks to the patients with high profile recalls [2]. Nearly 5,000 individual classes of medical devices, tens of thousands of medical device suppliers, and millions of healthcare providers exist worldwide, which clearly depicts that device-related issues are likely to occur. The outcome of an adverse event related to medical devices can be serious and result in illness, injury or even death, which have led experts to call for the monitoring of the safe and effective use of medical devices after its regulatory approval [3].

Materiovigilance Programme of India (MvPI) was launched in 2015 and has implemented a robust system to ensure the safety of medical devices. The aim of this programme is to identify the adverse events associated with the use of medical devices and to eliminate the device-related risks through a systematic reporting system [4]. In India, the Medical Devices Rules (MDR) were notified on January 31st, 2017 and became effective from January 1st, 2018. As per the MDR, G.S.R. 78 (E), Chapter 4, Section 26 (ii) "the License Holder shall inform the State Licensing Authority (SLA) or Central Licensing Authority (CLA), as the case may be of the occurrence of any suspected unexpected serious adverse events and take necessary action thereon, including any recall within 15 days of such event coming to the notice of License Holder" [5] (**Table 1**). The MDR, in concurrence with MvPI, has significantly influenced the post marketing surveillance of medical devices among the healthcare professionals, by ensuring their quality and patient/user safety [5]. This chapter aims to describe the systems, procedures and modalities available for the reporting of Medical Device Adverse Events (MDAEs) in India, in order to intensify the nature of reporting and creating an environment that encourages the public to perform MDAE reporting.

Reporter	What to report?	To Whom?	When?
Marketing Authorisation Holders (MAH)/Manufacturers/ Importers/Distributors	Any suspected unexpected serious adverse event incident, such as deaths, serious injuries, malfunction, etc., together with the action taken thereon, including any recall	National Regulatory body National Coordination Centre (NCC) – Indian Pharmacopeia Commission (IPC)	Within 15 calendar days after becoming aware of an event.
Healthcare professionals	Death, serious injuries, malfunction, etc.	National Regulatory body National Coordination Centre (NCC) – Indian Pharmacopeia Commission (IPC) Marketing Authorisation Holders (MAHs)	For serious events, the reporting has to be done within 15 calendar days after becoming aware of an event. For non-serious events, the reporting has to be done within 30 calendar days after becoming aware of an event.

Table 1.
Mandatory reporting requirements.

2. MvPI Focus Groups for MDAE reporting

The following groups play a significant role in the smooth functioning of MvPI:

2.1 Medical Device Adverse Event Monitoring Centres (MDMCs) and Adverse Drug Reactions Monitoring Centres (AMCs)

Healthcare facilities, including district/government/private hospitals, and autonomous bodies are recognized as MDMCs and AMCs by the NCC-MvPI, IPC and NCC-PvPI, IPC respectively. The function of the MDMC is to raise awareness about the programme and reporting of MDAEs. The MvPI collects reports from the MDMCs, AMCs. Under the MvPI, 50 MDMCs have been identified so far in India to collect the report of the events associated with the use of medical devices [6]. The AMCs established under the Pharmacovigilance Programme of India (PvPI) are also participating in MDAE reporting. Around 311 centres have been identified in the country to report the adverse events resulting from the use of drugs/medical products [7].

2.2 Medical device industries

Medical device industries, including manufacturers, importers, distributors, etc., are approached and encouraged to report the MDAE, particularly with their own medical devices. As there may be chances of re-occurrences of the adverse events, medical device industries play a key role in medical device safety surveillance [8].

2.3 Healthcare professionals

Healthcare facilities include healthcare professionals, such as clinical specialists, biomedical engineers, nurses, pharmacists, hospital technology managers, and technicians, as well as patients. Healthcare professionals are in direct contact both with the patients and the medical devices used in the healthcare facilities, and are hence the key personnel in MDAE reporting [9].

2.4 Accreditation bodies

Accreditation bodies essentially identify the capability of the hospitals to deliver quality care. Indian healthcare institutions get accreditation from bodies such as the National Accreditation Board for Hospitals and Healthcare providers (NABH). The IPC has signed a Memorandum of Understanding (MoU) with the NABH, under the Quality Council of India (QCI), to ensure for total cooperation of the hospitals on the reporting of adverse events associated with medical devices in the hospital [10].

3. Modalities for MDAE reporting

The NCC for MvPI, IPC has developed the below-mentioned reporting tools to collect MDAEs. All the reporting tools are available on the IPC website. The healthcare professionals, MAHs and all the Personal Protective Equipments (PPEs) users are encouraged to report adverse events associated with medical devices [11].

3.1 MDAE reporting form

The MDAE reporting form primarily aims to collect the adverse events associated with the use of medical devices, *In-Vitro* Diagnostics (IVDs), and medical equipments. The healthcare professionals and others including, but not limited to, manufacturers, importers, distributors, and hospital managers are solicited to report the adverse events for known, unknown, serious, non-serious, frequent or rare adverse events. The MDAE reporting form assembles adverse event information associated with medical devices and consists of the following nine sections (**Figure 1**) [11].

3.1.1 General information

This section includes the date of report, *i.e.* the date in which the report was filled, and the type of report that specifies whether the event is Initial/Follow-up/Final/Trend. The initial report is the first event notification report which may include the minimal required information, for instance, device information, details of adverse event and reporter details. A report may be marked as a follow-up report when additional information is available from the previously reported event. The report may be submitted as a final report when all the information associated with the event is available and collected. If the reporter is observing a significant number of similar adverse events, the reporter may tick the trend option [12].

3.1.2 Reporter details

This section comprises the type of reporter, along with the details of the reporter, including name, address, contact number and e-mail address. A reporter may be a manufacturer, importer, distributor, healthcare professional, patient, or other. The information provided in this section is kept confidential and only utilised for further follow-up.

3.1.3 Device category

This section refers to the general information about the medical device used. The device category section in the MDAE reporting form consists of three subsections, namely medical device, medical equipment and IVDs. The medical equipment and IVDs subsections refer to specific categories of medical devices. Medical devices requiring calibration, maintenance, repair, user training and decommissioning – are usually managed by clinical engineers. Medical equipment is used for the specific purposes of diagnosis and treatment of disease or rehabilitation following disease or injury. It can be used either alone or in combination with any accessory, consumable or other piece of medical equipment. Medical equipment excludes implantable, disposable or single-use medical devices. The IVD medical devices includes a medical device, used either alone or in combination, intended by the manufacturer for the *in-vitro* examination of specimens derived from the human body solely or principally to provide information for diagnostic, monitoring or compatibility purposes. All the other devices not covered under the definitions of medical equipments and IVDs should be included into the medical device subsection.

3.1.4 Device description

This section describes the specific details of the suspected medical device: device name or the brand name used for marketing of the device, manufacturing or import firm name and address, the information of local distributer, the lot/batch number,

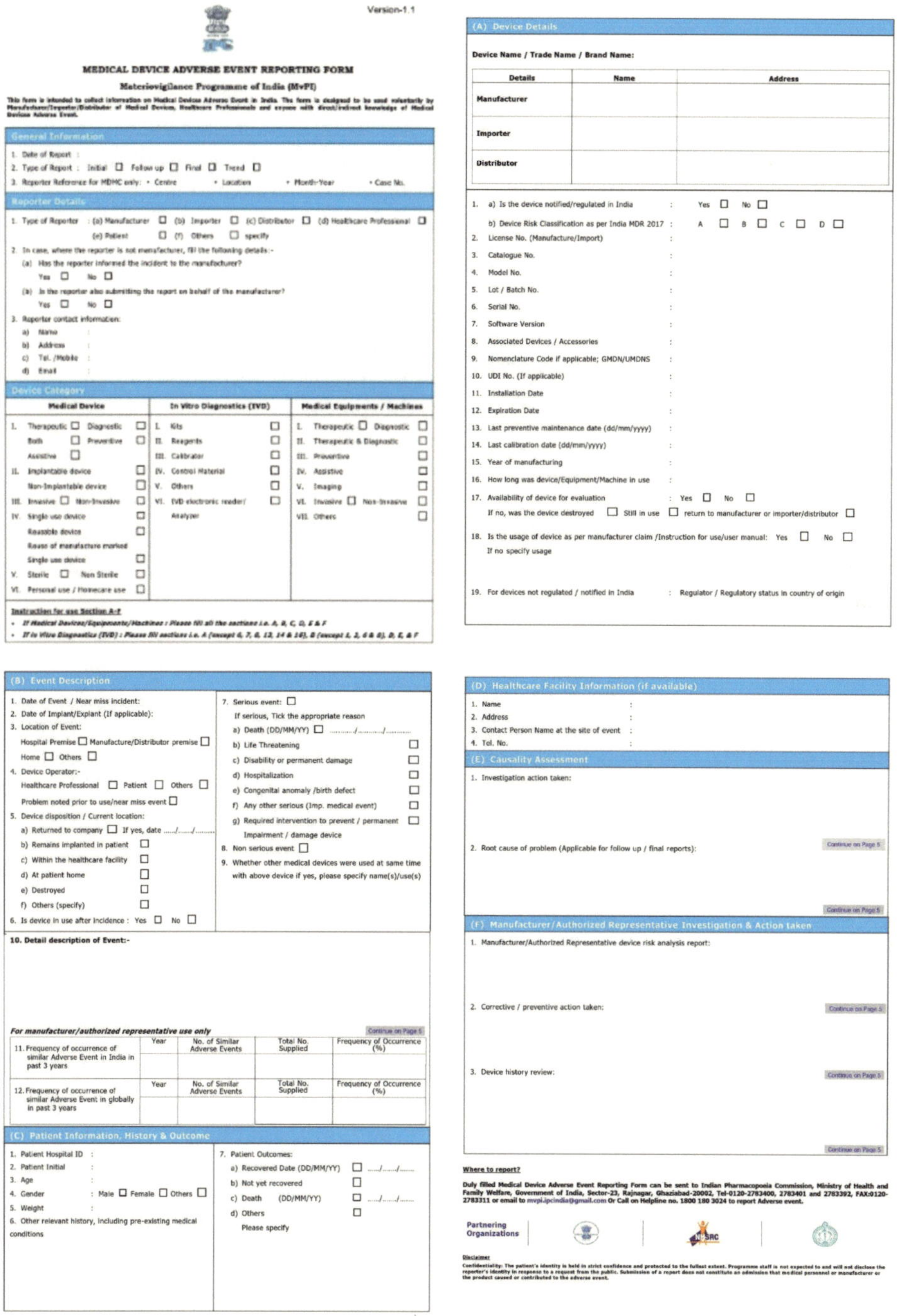

Version-1.1

MEDICAL DEVICE ADVERSE EVENT REPORTING FORM

Materiovigilance Programme of India (MvPI)

General Information

1. Date of Report :
2. Type of Report : Initial ☐ Follow up ☐ Final ☐ Trend ☐
3. Reporter Reference for MDMC only: • Centre • Location • Month-Year • Case No.

Reporter Details

1. Type of Reporter : (a) Manufacturer ☐ (b) Importer ☐ (c) Distributor ☐ (d) Healthcare Professional ☐ (e) Patient ☐ (f) Others ☐ specify
2. In case, where the reporter is not manufacturer, fill the following details :-
   (a) Has the reporter informed the incident to the manufacturer? Yes ☐ No ☐
   (b) Is the reporter also submitting the report on behalf of the manufacturer? Yes ☐ No ☐
3. Reporter contact information:
   a) Name :
   b) Address :
   c) Tel. /Mobile :
   d) Email :

Device Category

Medical Device	In Vitro Diagnostics (IVD)	Medical Equipments / Machines
I. Therapeutic ☐ Diagnostic ☐ Both ☐ Preventive ☐ Assistive ☐	I. Kits ☐	I. Therapeutic ☐ Diagnostic ☐
II. Implantable device ☐ Non-Implantable device ☐	II. Reagents ☐	II. Therapeutic & Diagnostic ☐
III. Invasive ☐ Non-Invasive ☐	III. Calibrator ☐	III. Preventive ☐
IV. Single use device ☐ Reusable device ☐ Reuse of manufacture marked Single use device ☐	IV. Control Material ☐	IV. Assistive ☐
V. Sterile ☐ Non Sterile ☐	V. Others ☐	V. Imaging ☐
VI. Personal use / Homecare use ☐	VI. IVD electronic reader/ Analyzer ☐	VI. Invasive ☐ Non-Invasive ☐
		VII. Others ☐

(A) Device Details

Device Name / Trade Name / Brand Name:

Details	Name	Address
Manufacturer		
Importer		
Distributor		

1. a) Is the device notified/regulated in India : Yes ☐ No ☐
   b) Device Risk Classification as per India MDR 2017 : A ☐ B ☐ C ☐ D ☐
2. License No. (Manufacture/Import) :
3. Catalogue No. :
4. Model No. :
5. Lot / Batch No. :
6. Serial No. :
7. Software Version :
8. Associated Devices / Accessories :
9. Nomenclature Code if applicable; GMDN/UMDNS :
10. UDI No. (If applicable) :
11. Installation Date :
12. Expiration Date :
13. Last preventive maintenance date (dd/mm/yyyy) :
14. Last calibration date (dd/mm/yyyy) :
15. Year of manufacturing :
16. How long was device/Equipment/Machine in use :
17. Availability of device for evaluation : Yes ☐ No ☐
    If no, was the device destroyed ☐ Still in use ☐ return to manufacturer or importer/distributor ☐
18. Is the usage of device as per manufacturer claim /Instruction for use/user manual: Yes ☐ No ☐
    If no specify usage
19. For devices not regulated / notified in India : Regulator / Regulatory status in country of origin

(B) Event Description

1. Date of Event / Near miss incident:
2. Date of Implant/Explant (If applicable):
3. Location of Event:
   Hospital Premise ☐ Manufacture/Distributor premise ☐ Home ☐ Others ☐
4. Device Operator:-
   Healthcare Professional ☐ Patient ☐ Others ☐
   Problem noted prior to use/near miss event ☐
5. Device disposition / Current location:
   a) Returned to company ☐ If yes, date ..../..../....
   b) Remains implanted in patient ☐
   c) Within the healthcare facility ☐
   d) At patient home ☐
   e) Destroyed ☐
   f) Others (specify) ☐
6. Is device in use after incidence : Yes ☐ No ☐
7. Serious event: ☐
   If serious, Tick the appropriate reason
   a) Death (DD/MM/YY) ☐ ..../..../....
   b) Life Threatening ☐
   c) Disability or permanent damage ☐
   d) Hospitalization ☐
   e) Congenital anomaly /birth defect ☐
   f) Any other serious (Imp. medical event) ☐
   g) Required intervention to prevent / permanent Impairment / damage device ☐
8. Non serious event ☐
9. Whether other medical devices were used at same time with above device if yes, please specify name(s)/use(s)

10. Detail description of Event:-

For manufacturer/authorized representative use only

	Year	No. of Similar Adverse Events	Total No. Supplied	Frequency of Occurrence (%)
11. Frequency of occurrence of similar Adverse Event in India in past 3 years				
12. Frequency of occurrence of similar Adverse Event in globally in past 3 years				

(C) Patient Information, History & Outcome

1. Patient Hospital ID :
2. Patient Initial :
3. Age :
4. Gender : Male ☐ Female ☐ Others ☐
5. Weight :
6. Other relevant history, including pre-existing medical conditions
7. Patient Outcomes:
   a) Recovered Date (DD/MM/YY) ☐ ..../..../....
   b) Not yet recovered ☐
   c) Death (DD/MM/YY) ☐ ..../..../....
   d) Others ☐
   Please specify

(D) Healthcare Facility Information (if available)

1. Name :
2. Address :
3. Contact Person Name at the site of event :
4. Tel. No. :

(E) Causality Assessment

1. Investigation action taken:
2. Root cause of problem (Applicable for follow up / final reports):

(F) Manufacturer/Authorized Representative Investigation & Action taken

1. Manufacturer/Authorized Representative device risk analysis report:
2. Corrective / preventive action taken:
3. Device history review:

Where to report?

Duly filled Medical Device Adverse Event Reporting Form can be sent to Indian Pharmacopoeia Commission, Ministry of Health and Family Welfare, Government of India, Sector-23, Rajnagar, Ghaziabad-20002, Tel-0120-2783400, 2783401 and 2783392, FAX:0120-2783311 or email to mvpi.ipcindia@gmail.com Or Call on Helpline no. 1800 180 3024 to report Adverse event.

Partnering Organizations

Disclaimer:

Figure 1.
Pictorial representation of medical device adverse event (MDAE) reporting form.

serial number, year of manufacturing. Furthermore, in case of medical equipment, the additional information also includes installation date, last calibration date and preventive maintenance date, and software version is also asked. Many countries use different nomenclature systems for naming the medical device. The most prominent codes known are the Global Medical Device Nomenclature (GMDN) and Universal Medical Device Nomenclature System (UMDNS). In the reporting form, the reporter has an option to add the nomenclature code of the device while reporting the event.

3.1.5 Event description

This section includes the most important dates associated with the adverse event, such as the date in which the event or any near miss incident occurred, etc. Furthermore, this section also comprises the information about device operator, device location and the detailed description of the event. The reporter may mark an event as serious in case it fulfils the seriousness criteria described in MDR 2017 [5]. Otherwise, the event may be marked as non-serious.

3.1.6 Patient information

This section contains the patient information, including its medical history and final patient outcome after the adverse event has occurred. Additionally, the patient hospital ID, age, gender is also comprised in this section.

3.1.7 Healthcare facility information

This section includes the details of the hospital in which the event took place, as well as the details of a contact person at the hospital, for the further follow-up communication related to the adverse event.

3.1.8 Causality assessment

This section aims to collect the information regarding the investigation process carried out by the clinical specialists from the healthcare facility, or by the concerned personnel from the manufacturing organization, to further drawing out the root cause of the problem and the immediate action taken to reverse the adverse effect, if possible. The root cause will ascertain the most likely reason for the occurrence of the adverse event.

3.1.9 Manufacturer/Authorized representative investigation & action taken

This section provides the information related to the investigation methods performed by the manufacturer/authorized representative and device history, which includes a review of similar events occurred from the same batch/lot, the analysis report of the event related to the medical device, and the corrective/preventive action/recall taken to prevent the patient from being affected by the device, if any. The MDAE form is designed in such a manner that it collects the maximum information required, which may be helpful for the identification of the MDAE and for creating the database of the medical device-related errors, thus enabling to trace the trend of adverse events associated with medical devices. The MDAE form may also help the medical device stakeholders to provide appropriate information and enhance the quality of the information collected.

3.2 PPE Reporting Form

During the prevailing situation regarding the COVID-19 pandemic, the NCC-MvPI specially designed a one-page editable MDAE reporting form, which primarily aims to collect the adverse events associated with the use of PPEs used for medical purposes (**Figure 2**) [11]. The information required to be filled in the reporting form under the different categories is as follows [11]:

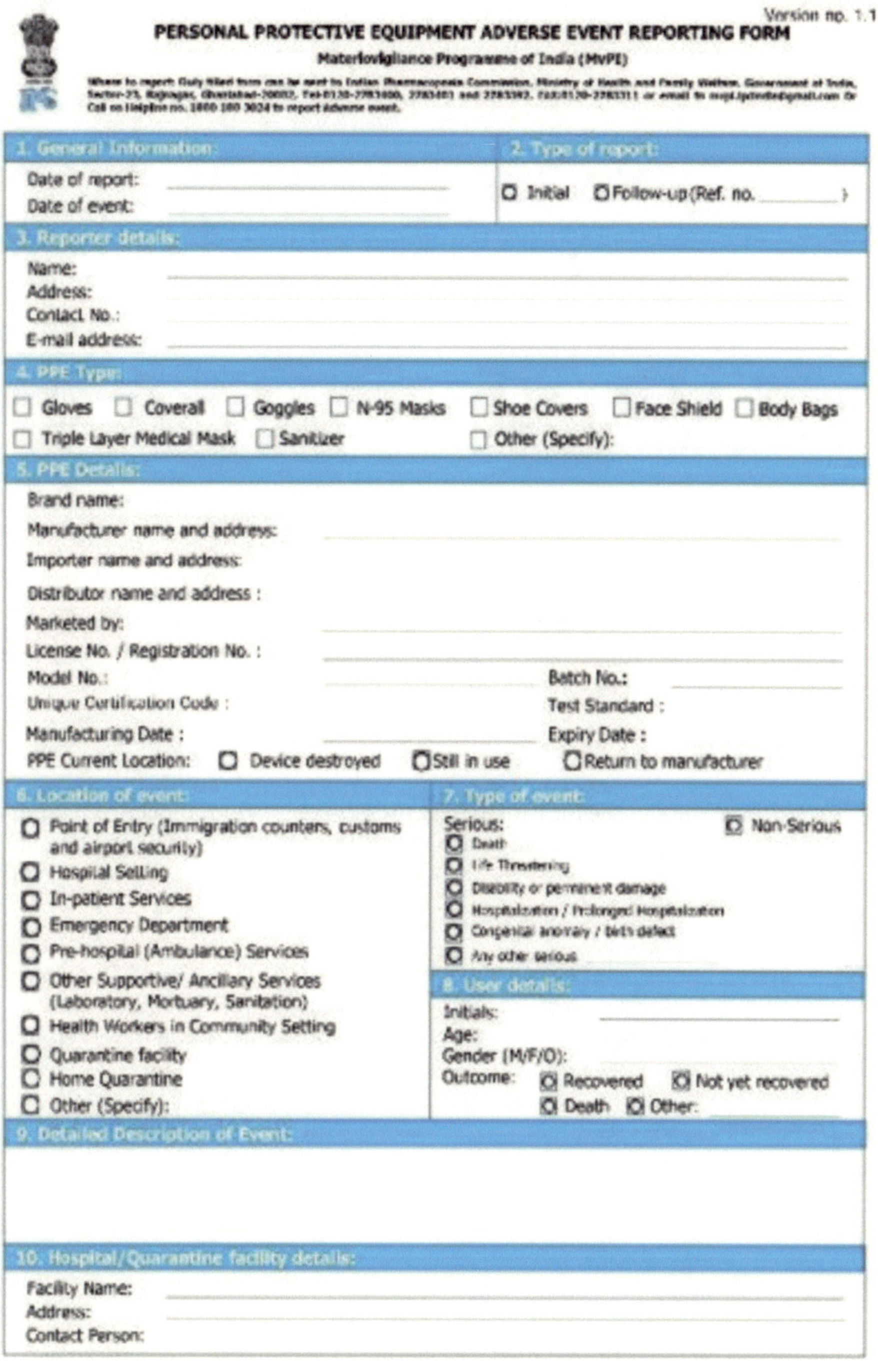

Version no. 1.1

PERSONAL PROTECTIVE EQUIPMENT ADVERSE EVENT REPORTING FORM

Materiovigilance Programme of India (MvPI)

Where to report: Duly filled form can be sent to Indian Pharmacopoeia Commission, Ministry of Health and Family Welfare, Government of India, Sector-23, Rajnagar, Ghaziabad-201002. Tel:0120-2783400, 2783401 and 2783392. Fax:0120-2783311 or email to mvpi.ipcindia@gmail.com Or Call on Helpline no. 1800 180 3024 to report Adverse event.

1. General Information:
Date of report:
Date of event:

2. Type of report:
Initial / Follow-up (Ref. no.)

3. Reporter details:
Name:
Address:
Contact No.:
E-mail address:

4. PPE Type:
Gloves / Coverall / Goggles / N-95 Masks / Shoe Covers / Face Shield / Body Bags / Triple Layer Medical Mask / Sanitizer / Other (Specify):

5. PPE Details:
Brand name:
Manufacturer name and address:
Importer name and address:
Distributor name and address :
Marketed by:
License No. / Registration No. :
Model No.: Batch No.:
Unique Certification Code : Test Standard :
Manufacturing Date : Expiry Date :
PPE Current Location: Device destroyed / Still in use / Return to manufacturer

6. Location of event:
Point of Entry (Immigration counters, customs and airport security)
Hospital Setting
In-patient Services
Emergency Department
Pre-hospital (Ambulance) Services
Other Supportive/ Ancillary Services (Laboratory, Mortuary, Sanitation)
Health Workers in Community Setting
Quarantine facility
Home Quarantine
Other (Specify):

7. Type of event:
Serious: Death / Life Threatening / Disability or permanent damage / Hospitalization / Prolonged Hospitalization / Congenital anomaly / birth defect / Any other serious
Non-Serious

8. User details:
Initials:
Age:
Gender (M/F/O):
Outcome: Recovered / Not yet recovered / Death / Other:

9. Detailed Description of Event:

10. Hospital/Quarantine facility details:
Facility Name:
Address:
Contact Person:

Figure 2.
Pictorial representation of personal protective equipment (PPE) reporting form.

3.2.1 General information

This section includes the exact date in which the event was reported to the NCC-MvPI, IPC, and the type of report that specifies whether the event is Initial/Follow-up. The initial report is the first notification about an adverse event submitted to the NCC-MvPI, IPC, once the reporter became aware of it. The follow-up report comprises the additional information about the previous report.

3.2.2 Reporter details

This section comprises the details of the reporter, including name, address, contact number and e-mail address. The information provided in this section is kept confidential and only utilized for the follow-up.

3.2.3 PPE type

This section encompasses the type of PPE involved in the adverse event/reaction-gloves, coverall, goggles, N-95 masks, shoe covers, face shields, body bags, triple layer medical mask, among others.

3.2.4 PPE details

This section describes the specific details of the PPE involved in the adverse event. These details include the brand name, manufacturer/importer/distributer name, batch number, model number, license number, unique certification code, test standard followed, manufacturing date and expiry date.

3.2.5 Location of event

This section refers to the location where the adverse event has occurred, and includes inpatient department, quarantine facilities, emergency department, etc.

3.2.6 Type of event

This section comprises the seriousness of the event. If the event involves the following outcomes: death/life threatening/disability or permanent damage/hospitalization/congenital anomaly, then it should be marked as serious. Otherwise, the event may be marked as non-serious.

3.2.7 User details

This section covers the details of the PPE user, including user initials, age, gender, etc.

3.2.8 Event description

This section includes the detailed description of an adverse event associated with PPEs.

3.2.9 Hospital/quarantine facility details

This section provides the details related to the hospital/quarantine facilities, including name, address and contact person. The PPE form is designed in such a manner that it collects all the required information, which may be used for the identification of PPE-related adverse events and for creating the database of such adverse events.

3.3 Field safety corrective action (FSCA) notification form

The FSCA [11] refers to any action taken to reduce a risk of death or serious deterioration in the state of health associated with the use of a medical device, including the: (i) device returned to the manufacturer, (ii) device design changes, (iii) device software upgrade, (iv) labelling changes, (v) changes in instructions for use or directions for use or technical manual, (vi) device destruction and (vii) device exchange. For more information, see [13].

3.4 Legal obligation

The submitted MDAE report does not have any legal implication concerning the reporters. The patients' identity will be held under strict confidence and protected to its full extent. As the reporting programme is voluntary in nature, healthcare providers are encouraged to report adverse events for a better understanding of the risk associated with the use of medical devices, and to safeguard the health of the Indian population [14].

3.5 Essential data for effective reporting

This section includes the following information: date of event, reporter contact information, device name, manufacturer/importer/distributor details, catalogue number., lot/batch number., serial number., model number., date of implantation/explantation (if applicable), seriousness of the event, event description, patient history, patient outcome, healthcare facility information, root cause and corrective/preventive action [13].

3.6 Factors contributing to a serious adverse event

The improper functioning of the medical devices, manufacturing defects, design and labelling issues, user and procedural errors are some examples of the major contributing factors that can lead to the occurrence of a serious adverse event if underestimated [15].

4. Helpline facility for reporting adverse events

The IPC has already launched a toll-free helpline facility, helpline Number- 1800 180 3024 (Monday to Friday- 9:00 am to 5:30 pm), for the reporting of adverse drug reactions by healthcare professionals and others [16]. Currently, this facility is also being extended to the report of any adverse event associated with the use of medical devices. Both the data management and the procedure adopted to receive the information from the healthcare professionals, patients and others are given in **Figure 3**.

5. Enrolment process as MDMC under MvPI

Healthcare facilities including district/government/private hospitals, and autonomous bodies are recognized as MDMCs and AMCs respectively by the NCC-MvPI, IPC and NCC-PvPI, IPC. The function of MDMC is to raise awareness about the programme and reporting of MDAEs. A 'Letter of Intent' is required to be submitted by the head of the Institution/hospital for participating in this nationwide programme to

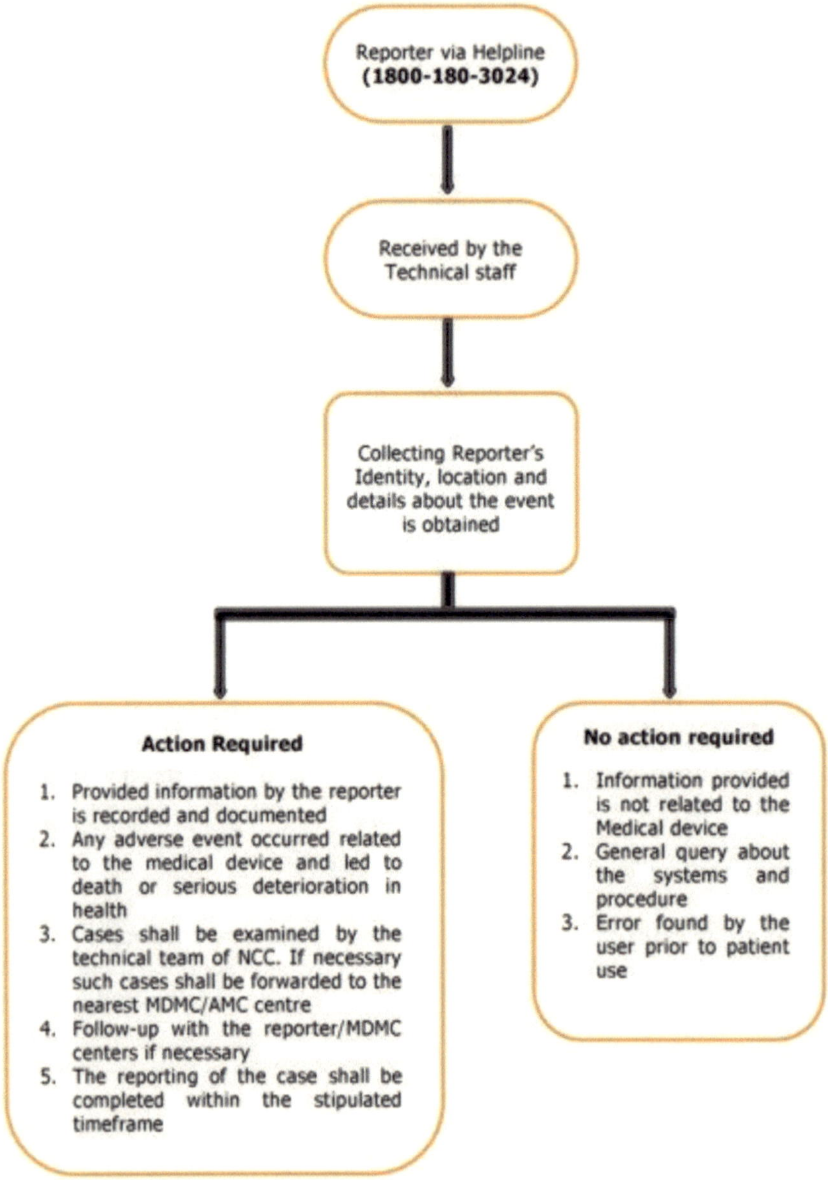

Figure 3.
Flow diagram representing the report of adverse events related to medical devices through helpline.

monitor MDAEs [17]. After the suitability examination by the competent authority, the proposed centre may be recognized as an MDMC under MvPI. These centres are expected to collate data on adverse events associated with medical devices and IVDs under the MvPI and report them to the NCC-MvPI, IPC. For the proper functioning of MvPI activities in their respective centres, a research associate will be appointed by the NCC-MvPI, IPC [18]. The research associate will be responsible for the collection of reports and conduction of training programs on materiovigilance, aiming to sensitize the healthcare professionals and the general public. The technical team at the MDMC performs the validation of the report by carrying out the causality assessment to identify any causal/temporal relationship between the event and the medical device. The workflow for determining the report responsible for the identification of adverse events significantly related to medical devices is shown at **Figure 4**.

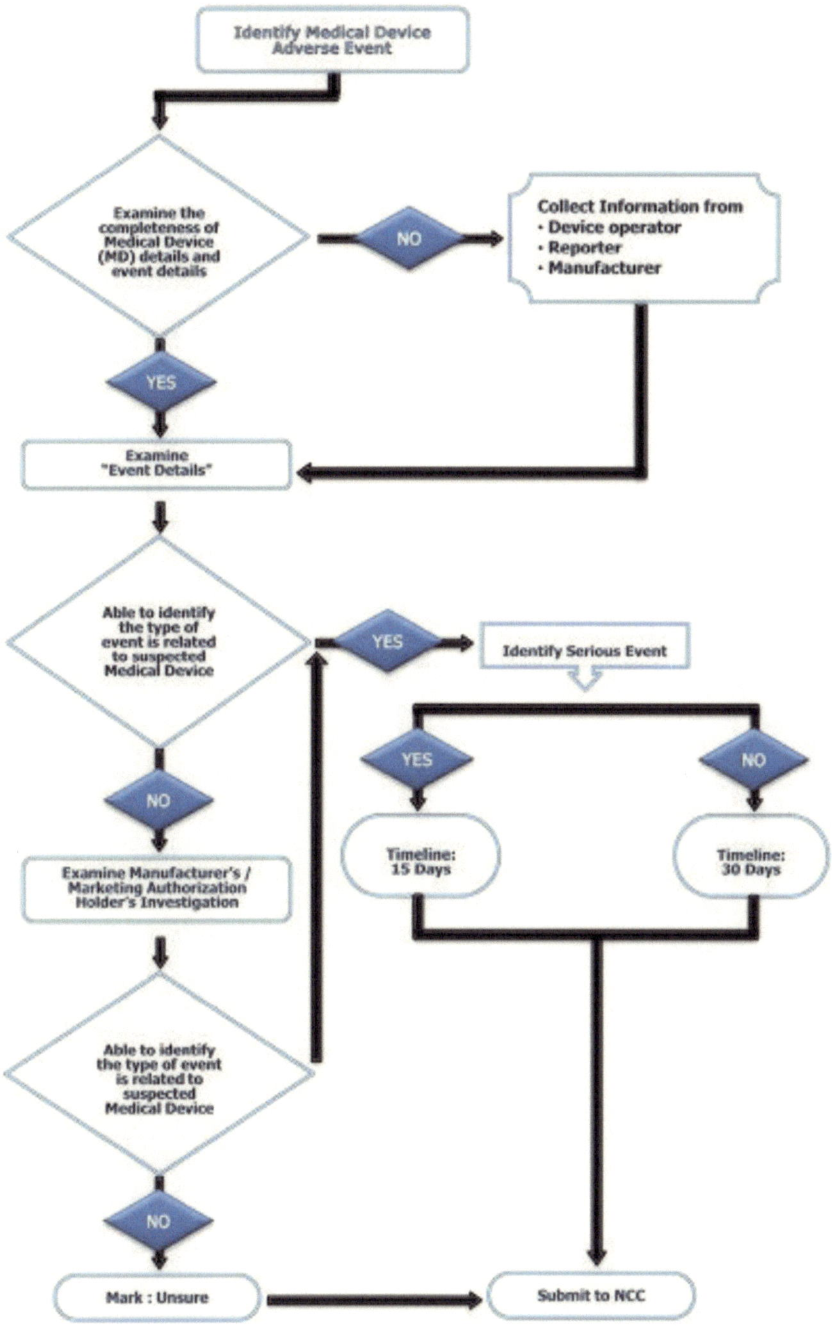

Figure 4.
Medical device-related adverse events identification flowchart used at medical device adverse event monitoring centres (MDMC).

6. Report Handling and Management

Initially, the reports are collected and analysed at the NCC-MvPI, IPC, by applying the globally recognized scientific standards/parameters to ensure the quality of the reports. In the second level, these analysed cases are forwarded to the subject expert group panel for review, and technical interpretation is drawn considering both the clinical, as well as technical aspects. In the third level, these reports are placed before the core technical committee for the conclusions and recommendations, and are further forwarded to the national regulatory authority for implementation of the necessary actions (**Figure 4**) [19].

7. Data Generated

The NCC has collected the reported adverse events and provided a comparison of the serious adverse events reported in the index period from January to December during the years of 2018, 2019 and 2020. In total, NCC has received 3187 adverse events, consisting of 1986 serious and 1201 non-serious events. Out of the serious adverse events reported, 23% were reported in 2018, 37% in 2019 and 40% in 2020. When comparing the reported data, an increase of 75% in serious adverse event reporting could be observed. Out of the adverse events reported, 73% of the reports were received from MAHs, 23% from MDMCs and 4% from AMCs [19]. This confirms and highlights the importance of the modalities developed, as they have significantly helped to improve the reporting of adverse events related to medical devices.

8. Conclusion

The tools developed for reporting may stimulate the communication between medical device users and the regulatory authorities to closely monitor medical device safety. In order to generate proper regulatory decisions and to ensure the quality and efficacy of the medical devices that are being sold and distributed in the Indian market, MvPI has shown to provide a robust and sustainable system for collecting and reporting adverse events associated with medical devices. This will highly encourage all the healthcare professionals, MAH and the public to efficiently report adverse events associated with medical devices.

Acknowledgements

The authors are grateful to Ministry of Health & Family Welfare, Government of India for the financial support provided to run the MvPI efficiently.

Conflict of interest statement

The authors declare no potential conflict of interest.

Abbreviations

AMC	Adverse Drug Reaction Monitoring Centre
CLA	Central Licensing Authority
FSCA	Field Safety Corrective Action
FSN	Field Safety Notice
GMDN	Global Medical Device Nomenclature
IPC	Indian Pharmacopoeia Commission
IVDs	*In-Vitro* Diagnostics

MAH	Marketing Authorisation Holders
MDAE	Medical Device Adverse Event
MDMC	Medical Device Adverse Event Monitoring Centre
MDR	Medical Device Rules
MoU	Memorandum of Understanding
MvPI	Materiovigilance Programme of India
NABH	National Accreditation Board for Hospitals and Healthcare providers
NCC	National Coordination Centre
PPE	Personal Protective Equipment
PvPI	Pharmacovigilance Programme of India
QCI	Quality Council of India
SEARN	South East Asia Research Network
SLA	State Licensing Authority
UDI	Unique Device Identification
UMDN	Universal Medical Device Nomenclature

Author details

Vivekanandan Kalaiselven*, Shatrunajay Shukla, Nikita Mishra and Pawan Kumar
Materiovigilance Associate in Materiovigilance Programme of India, Indian Pharmacopoeia Commission, Ministry of Health and Family Welfare, Government of India, Ghaziabad, Uttar Pradesh, India

*Address all correspondence to: vivekarts@rediffmail.com

References

[1] Materiovigilance and Medical Devices, doi.org/10.1007/978-3-319-07653-9_21 [Online]. Available: https://link.springer.com/chapter/10.1007/978-3-319-07653-9_21 (accessed Mar. 15, 2021).

[2] Medical Device Recalls, FDA, Sep. 09, 2020. [Online]. Available: https://www.fda.gov/medical-devices/medical-device-safety/medical-device-recalls (accessed Feb. 24, 2021).

[3] Analysis of FDA-Approved Orthopaedic Devices and Their Recalls, JBJS, vol. 98, no. 6, pp. 517-524, Mar. 2016, doi: 10.2106/JBJS.15.00286 [Online]. Available: https://pubmed.ncbi.nlm.nih.gov/26984921/ (accessed Feb. 24, 2021).

[4] Materiovigilance programme of India (MvPI): A step towards patient safety for medical devices. [Online]. Available: https://www.researchgate.net/publication/338065787_MATERIO VIGILANCE_PROGRAMME_OF_INDIA_MvPI_A_STEP_TOWARDS_PATIENT_SAFETY_FOR_MEDICAL_DEVICES (accessed Feb. 24, 2021).

[5] Medical device rules 2017, [Online]. Available: https://cdsco.gov.in/opencms/resources/UploadCDSCOWeb/2018/UploadGazette_NotificationsFiles/MedicalDeviceRulegsr78E.pdf (accessed Feb. 24, 2021).

[6] Materiovigilance: Current status in India analogous to its global status, DOI:10.5281/zenodo.4299028 [Online]. Available: https://zenodo.org/record/4299028#.YE9F0NIzZ0w.html (accessed Mar. 15, 2021).

[7] Pharmacovigilance Programme of India (PvPI) Updates - Indian Pharmacopoeia Commission, [Online]. Available: https://ipc.gov.in/mandates/pvpi/pvpi-updates.html (accessed Feb. 24, 2021).

[8] Implementation of adverse event reporting for medical devices, India, [Online]. Available: https://www.researchgate.net/publication/339488352_Implementation_of_adverse_event_reporting_for_medical_devices_India (accessed Feb. 24, 2021).

[9] MATERIOVIGILANCE: AN EMERGING DISCIPLINE [Online]. Available: https://www.worldwide journals.com/international-journal-of-scientific-research (IJSR)/fileview.php?val=June_2018_1527932925__36.pdf (accessed Mar. 15, 2021).

[10] Pivotal role of Pharmacovigilance Programme of India in containment of antimicrobial resistance in India, doi: 10.4103/picr.PICR_29_18 [Online]. Available: https://www.ncbi.nlm.nih.gov/pmc/articles/PMC6647896/ (accessed Feb. 24, 2021).

[11] Medical Devices Adverse Event Reporting Tools - Indian Pharmacopoeia Commission [Online]. Available: https://ipc.gov.in/mandates/pvpi/materiovigilance-programme-of-india-mvpi.html?id=597:medical-devices-adverse-event-reporting-tools&catid=2 (accessed Feb. 24, 2021).

[12] Adverse events reporting of medical devices, HSA. [Online]. Available: https://www.hsa.gov.sg/medical-devices/adverse-events (accessed Feb. 24, 2021).

[13] Guidance Document: Materiovigilance Programme of India (version 1.2). [Online]. Available: https://ipc.gov.in/images/Guideline_-_11-03-2020.pdf (accessed Feb. 24, 2021).

[14] Materiovigilance: An Indian perspective, Perspect Clin Res, vol. 9, no. 4, pp. 175-178, 2018, doi: 10.4103/picr.PICR_26_18. [Online]. Available: https://pubmed.ncbi.nlm.nih.gov/30319948/ (accessed Feb. 24, 2021).

[15] Medical Device Reporting (MDR): How to Report Medical Device Problems, FDA, Oct. 05, 2020. https://www.fda.gov/medical-devices/medical-device-safety/medical-device-reporting-mdr-how-report-medical-device-problems (accessed Feb. 24, 2021).

[16] V. Kalaiselvan, P. Mishra, and G. N. Singh, "Helpline facility to assist reporting of adverse drug reactions in India," WHO South East Asia J Public Health, vol. 3, no. 2, p. 194, Jun. 2014, doi: 10.4103/2224-3151.206737[Online]. Available: https://pubmed.ncbi.nlm.nih.gov/28607307/(accessed Feb. 24, 2021).

[17] Letter of Intent for enrolling as medical device adverse event monitoring center under materiovigilance programme. [Online]. Available: https://ipc.gov.in/images/pdf/File715.pdf (accessed Feb. 24, 2021).

[18] Materiovigilance Programme of India, DOI: 10.5958/0974-360X.2021.00204.3 – An Overview. [Online]. Available: https://rjptonline.org/HTMLPaper.aspx?Journal=Research%20Journal%20of%20Pharmacy%20and%20Technology; PID=2021-14-2-100 (accessed Mar. 15, 2021).

[19] S. Shukla et al., "Implementation of adverse event reporting for medical devices, India," Bull World Health Organ, vol. 98, no. 3, pp. 206-211, Mar. 2020, doi: 10.2471/BLT.19.232785. [Online]. Available: https://apps.who.int/iris/handle/10665/331375 (accessed Feb. 24, 2021).